Soul Matters – The Spiritual Dimension within Healthcare

Soul Matters – The Spiritual Dimension within Healthcare

MABEL AGHADIUNO

MB ChB DGM MRCGP MFHom MSc

Foreword by

CHRISTOPHER DOWRICK

BA MSc MD CQSW FRCGP FFPHM
Professor of Primary Medical Care
University of Liverpool

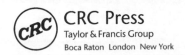

CRC Press
Taylor & Francis Group
Boca Raton London New York

CRC Press is an imprint of the
Taylor & Francis Group, an **informa** business

Radcliffe Publishing Ltd
18 Marcham Road
Abingdon
Oxon OX14 1AA
United Kingdom

www.radcliffe-oxford.com

Electronic catalogue and worldwide online ordering facility.

British Library Cataloguing in Publication Data

A catalogue record for this book is available from the British Library.

ISBN-13: 978 184619 166 4

The paper used for the text pages of this book
is FSC certified. FSC (The Forest Stewardship
Council) is an international network to promote
responsible management of the world's forests.

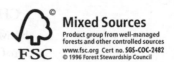

Mixed Sources
Product group from well-managed
forests and other controlled sources
www.fsc.org Cert no. SGS-COC-2482
© 1996 Forest Stewardship Council

Typeset by Phoenix Photosetting, Chatham, Kent

Contents

Foreword

Spirituality is the neglected cousin of healthcare. Health professionals are generally good at finding out what is wrong with people's physical health, and often not bad at helping people with psychological and emotional problems. We can sometimes identify the social and cultural dimensions of our patients' problems, but that is usually about as far as we go. When it comes to questions about meaning and purpose, such as 'what is the point of all this?', or 'why is this happening to me?', when we meet patients in the depths of despair at the prospect of imminent death, when we ourselves feel hopeless and overwhelmed in the face of an avalanche of human suffering, then we begin to struggle. We do not know what we could do, nor even what we should do. Our professional training doesn't help. We are stuck.

With this beautiful book, Mabel Aghadiuno comes to our rescue. Drawing on a wonderful diversity of sources, including literature and the arts, recent research and – above all – patient narratives and her own clinical experience, she elegantly explores the intricate connections between spirituality and healthcare. For Aghadiuno, we are all spiritual beings, and our spirituality is essentially a quest for meaning and transcendence: glimpses of which may be found equally in Messiaen's 'Quartet for the End of Time' or in the writings of Jacqueline du Pré. She explains how a sense of spirituality may pervade all aspects of medicine and healthcare, including mental health and complementary medicine, she advises us on how to undertake spiritual assessments, and she confronts head-on the thorny issues of despair and spiritual distress. Aghadiuno reminds us to acknowledge our role as healers, a concept that has fallen into decline and even disrepute in these days of evidence-based and policy-driven healthcare. And finally, through the moving account of the life and illnesses of Chiara M, she encourages us to retain hope in the face of adversity, and savour the transcendent to be found in living every day.

Christopher Dowrick
BA MSc MD CQSW FRCGP FFPHM
Professor of Primary Medical Care
University of Liverpool
November 2009

About the author

Dr Mabel Aghadiuno has been a General Practitioner (GP) for several years and is currently working for Lewisham Primary Care Trust in London. She graduated at Glasgow University and has worked in General Practice in Glasgow, Merseyside and London. She has been practising homeopathic medicine for some years and is on the specialist register of the Faculty of Homeopathy. Despite the seeming paradox, both conventional and homeopathic medicine sit comfortably with her. In 2003, her essay won the John Fry Bursary prize of the Royal Society of Medicine. Mabel is particularly interested in the art of medical practice.

Acknowledgements

I am most grateful to Chiara M for allowing me to use extracts of her writings and diary in Chapter 6. I am also very grateful for Lau Hung's permission to use the photographs of his sculptures which illustrate each chapter. Diane Godden and Joanna Carter's comments on the manuscript were very helpful.

I am especially thankful to patients, family, friends and colleagues who were the inspiration behind the writing of this book.

For permission to reprint copyright material and to use illustrations, the author and publisher gratefully acknowledge the following:

- Araujo V, Castellano J, Cola S, *et al. Dio Amore nella tradizione Cristiana e nella domanda dell'uomo contemporaneo.* Città Nuova Editrice; 1992. Reproduced with the kind permission of the publisher.
- Bridger F. *A Charmed Life: the spirituality of Potterworld.* Darton, Longman & Todd; 2001. Reproduced with the kind permission of the publisher.
- Campo R. 'Technology and Medicine'. In: *The Other Man Was Me.* Arte Publico Press, University of Houston; 1994. Reproduced with the kind permission of the publisher.
- Chiara M. *Crudele, dolcissimo amore.* Edizioni San Paolo; 2005. Reproduced with the kind permission of the author and publisher.
- Chiara M. *Oscura, luminosissima notte.* Edizioni San Paolo; 2008. Reproduced with the kind permission of the author and publisher.
- Coles R. *The Spiritual Life of Children.* Continuum International Publishing Group; 1990. Reproduced with the kind permission of the publisher.
- Coulehan J. 'Irene'. In: *The Knitted Glove.* Nightshade Press; 1991. Reproduced with the kind permission of the author.
- Dayton K. 'Procedures'. In: Haddad AM, Brown KH, editors. *The Arduous Touch: Women's Voices in Health Care.* Purdue University Press; 1999. Reproduced with the kind permission of the publisher.
- Excerpt from *Illness as Metaphor.* © 1977, 1978 Susan Sontag. Reprinted with the kind permission of Farrar, Straus and Giroux, LLC.
- Excerpt from the *New Jerusalem Bible.* Darton, Longman & Todd; 1995. Reproduced with the kind permission of the publisher.
- *FICA Questionnaire.* © Christina Puchalski, George Washington Institute for Spirituality and Health, www.gwish.org. Reproduced with kind permission.

- Foresi P. *Conversazioni di filosofia*. Città Nuova Editrice; 2001. Reproduced with the kind permission of the publisher.
- Frank A. *Wounded Storyteller: body, illness and ethics*. University of Chicago Press; 1997. Reproduced with the kind permission of the publisher.
- Fynn. *Anna and Mister God*. HarperCollins; 2004.
- Fynn. *Mister God, this is Anna*. William Co; 1974.
- Gurney I. 'To God'. In: *Collected Poems*. © Carcanet Press; 2004. Reproduced with the kind permission of the publisher.
- *Handbook for the Inspection of Schools*. © Office of Public Sector Information. Reproduced with kind permission.
- Hardy A. *Spiritual Nature of Man*. Oxford University Press; 1979. Reproduced with the kind permission of the publisher.
- *Herth Hope Index*. © 1989 Kaye Herth. Reproduced with the kind permission of the author.
- Kafka F. *Metamorphosis* (translated by Malcolm Pasley). Penguin Classics; 2000. Red Classics; 2006. Reproduced with the kind permission of the publisher.
- Kitwood T. *Dementia Reconsidered*. Open University Press; 1997. Reproduced with the kind permission of the publisher.
- Kliewer S, Saultz J. *Healthcare and Spirituality*. Radcliffe Publishing; 2006. Reproduced with the kind permission of the publisher.
- Klitzman R. *When Doctors Become Patients*. Oxford University Press; 2008. Reproduced with the kind permission of the publisher.
- Lewis CS. *Mere Christianity*. © 1942, 1943, 1944, 1952 CS Lewis Pte Ltd. Extract reproduced with permission.
- Lewis CS. *The Problem of Pain*. © 1940 CS Lewis Pte Ltd. Extract reproduced with permission.
- Lewis CS. *The Weight of Glory*. © 1949 CS Lewis Pte Ltd. Extract reproduced with permission.
- Morris T. *Philosophy for Dummies*. © John Wiley & Sons. Reproduced with the kind permission of the publisher.
- Paloutzian R, Ellison C. *Spiritual Well-Being Scale (SWB Scale)*. © Paloutzian, Ellison. Reproduced with kind permission.
- Pascal B. *Pensées* (translated with an introduction by AJ Krailsheimer). Penguin Classics; 1966. Reproduced with the kind permission of the publisher.
- Pellegrino ED, Thomasma DC. *Virtues in Medical Practice*. Oxford University Press; 2003. Reproduced with the kind permission of the publisher.
- *Promoting and evaluating pupils' spiritual, moral, social and cultural development*. © Office of Public Sector Information. Reproduced with kind permission.

- Schlaegel, TF, Jr. *Psychosomatic Ophthalmology.* William & Wilkins; 1957. Reproduced with the kind permission of the publisher.
- Smith T. *Homoeopathic Medicine for Mental Health.* Healing Arts Press; 1989. Reproduced with the kind permission of the publisher.
- *Sofferenza, malattia e morte nell'Africa sub-sahariana: prospettive per l'inculturazione N.3.* © 2005 Centro per l'inculturation. Extract translated by the author.
- Sontag S. *Illness as Metaphor.* The Penguin Group; 1983. Reproduced with the kind permission of the publisher.
- *Spirituality and Mental Health.* © Royal College of Psychiatrists. Extract reproduced with permission.
- Tolstoy L. *Anna Karenina* (translated with an introduction by Rosemary Edmonds). Penguin Books; 1954. Reproduced with the kind permission of the publisher.
- Torrance R. *The Spiritual Quest: transcendence in myth, religion and science.* University of California Press; 1994. Reproduced with the kind permission of the publisher.
- Ulz E. *L'uomo è l'artefice della sua vita.* Città Nuova Editrice; 2005. Reproduced with the kind permission of the publisher.
- Watts D. 'ms'. In: *Taking the History.* Nightshade Press; 1999. Reproduced with the kind permission of the author.
- Woolf V. *Moments of Being.* © The Society of Authors. Extract printed with permission.
- Zattoni M, Gillini G. *When Children Suffer Through Conflicts, Suffering & Loss* (translated by Simon Knight). Many Rooms Publishing; 2002. First published in 2000 in Italian as *Proteggere il Bambino.* Reproduced with the kind permission of the publisher.

I dedicate this book to everyone who has contributed – above all the silent heroes who grace hospital wards, wait patiently in doctors' surgeries and never fail to touch my life.

Introduction

THE SPIRITUAL DIMENSION OF HEALTH

Health is one of the hardest things to define. Roget's Thesaurus contains a plethora of words synonymous with health, some definitions being 'physical well-being' and 'bloom'. In Greek mythology, Hygeia was the ancient goddess of health. She was the daughter of Asclepius and is represented as a blooming maid with a bowl in her hand, from which she feeds a snake. The picture of health however varies from age to age. In Edwardian times a plump, rosy-cheeked woman would have epitomised health while in our day – at least in the West – advertisements portray the model woman: slim, attractive, 'flawless' and wrinkleless. The BBC website views health as a broader concept that includes being free from and resilient to disease, mental and spiritual wellbeing and the quality of our social relationships.[1] Instead the Australian Aborigines have an even wider perspective of health because for them it does not just mean the physical well-being of the individual but refers to the social, emotional, spiritual and cultural well-being of the whole community.[2] It is interesting what people will do in pursuit of health in the UK: eat tons of daily vitamin capsules, submit to coffee enemas, go on strict elimination diets and spend lots of money.

As with popular culture, within the scientific community the definition of health has evolved though perhaps not so equivocally. Over half a century ago WHO defined health as 'a complete state of physical, mental and social well-being, and not merely the absence of disease or infirmity'. There have been other definitions since then such as Bircher's[3] describing it as a 'dynamic state of well-being characterised by physical and mental potential, which satisfies the demands of life commensurate with age, culture and personal responsibility'. Cottrell *et al*[4] state that health requires a degree of balance among its varied dimensions that are physical, emotional, intellectual, social and spiritual. Butler[5] observes that the condition of one dimension often affects the condition of the other.

Butler's voice is not the sole one declaiming a link between the different dimensions of health. Hawks is the author of a stimulating article[6] where he says that health educators have inherited a preoccupation with physical health as the most laudable outcome of most of our programmes even though other dimensions of health seem equally important and even essential to the overall well-being of health programme participants. He argues spiritual health is an underlying dimension that contributes to social and emotional health. This in turn provides motivation for health behaviour changes that determine physical and intellectual health. Hawks stresses that a one-dimensional, segmented approach to health is inconsistent with our advocacy of holistic health promotion and that we run amiss if we promote physical health without addressing the other dimensions of health in a truly integrative model.

Therefore, it seems that in Western medicine, health professionals have lost contact with the spiritual health of patients. In the past, the same individual performed the role of the doctor and priest. In other cultures, this is still the case. Such a person is the shaman. The term shamanism comes from the Manchu-Tungus word *šaman*. The noun is formed from the verb ša-, 'to know'; thus, shaman literally means 'he who knows'. The shaman is believed to have direct contact through an ecstatic state with the transcendent world that permits him to act as healer, diviner, and escort of souls to the other world.

However, an attempt is being made to recover this lost, spiritual aspect and doctors do not need to be shamans to do this. A search on spiritual health of the WHO website gives 2300 hits. In fact, WHO has now broadened its definition of health by incorporating the spiritual dimension. It does however acknowledge that there are difficulties inherent in adopting such an approach. WHO points out that the Newtonian and Cartesian paradigm, characterised by a reductionist and materialist world-view, has dominated scientific thought. The spiritual dimension instead is an aspect of life belonging to a 'different paradigm of thought with entirely different ontological and epistemological assumptions'. WHO concludes that the spiritual dimension is an 'emergent property of a complex living system and exists only when such a system is examined in a holistic manner'.[7]

Puchalski and Larson[8] write that in recent years, patients and some members of the medical community have expressed the concern that doctors have forgotten about compassion and too often ignore their patients' spiritual concerns. They advocate medical schools have the duty to teach their students how to meet these expectations and that healthcare systems need to provide environments that 'foster compassionate care giving'.

Puchalski[9] illustrates this need to address the spiritual concerns of patients by giving a practical example. She relates the story of a HIV patient who refused treatment because she felt she had brought the condition on herself and that it was God's punishment. On taking a spiritual history, Puchalski was able to address her concerns by referring her to a trained chaplain. Puchalski also points out that there is a high burn out rate among doctors who want to be good at diagnosis and managing patients' illness and yet they still would like to give something more. She concludes that considering a patient's spiritual dimension would help fill this need to give the maximum to our patients.

Not all doctors agree with Puchalski. Sloan and several co-authors challenge the validity of studies that suggest religious activities support health, saying that such studies contain serious methodological flaws, conflicting findings, and data that lack clarity and specificity. Sloan goes on to suggest that when a physician addresses spirituality or religion with a patient, the potential exists for doing more harm than good. He agrees that there is a need to teach future physicians how to treat their patients as whole human beings rather than collections of organs, systems, and tissues. However, he says, a patient's spirituality is just one of many aspects in his or her life that influence behaviour and should not be singled out.[10, 11]

Whether or not we agree about the nature of the impact of the spiritual dimension on health, at least we should be able to recognise when it features in a case. I remember once seeing a patient with a very complicated domestic situation. He was in a complex dilemma and had some vague, non-specific symptoms that simply did not 'add up'. I then realised that his problem was not primarily physical but that it was essentially emotional and spiritual. I asked him if he practised any religion – thinking that it might be better for him to see a minister. He told me that he was 'RC, an atheist and what do I need to see one of them [a priest] for if I have got you, doctor?' Whether we like it or not some patients consciously or subconsciously do expect us to recognise and address what are often underlying spiritual problems. Sometimes we fail to recognise them as such, over-investigate and 'over-medicalise'.

Nonetheless, is the term 'spiritual dimension' not rather woolly and ill defined – if such a thing exists at all? In 1986 Sir Alister Hardy, naturalist and zoologist, did a study to help clarify if people have a spiritual nature. He examined the religious accounts of 1800 people and concluded that there was no doubt that the person has a spiritual nature. He describes it as that side of his make-up which might not necessarily lead to religious feelings, but at least gives a love of the non-material things of life such as natural beauty, art, music or moral values. Hardy observes that the spiritual side of the person is not the 'product of intellectuality' despite the fact that the development of the mind, so strongly prejudiced by scientific achievement, has tended to dismiss, as 'childish wishful thinking', this deeper property of life.[12]

Writing in *American Family Physician*, Anandarajah and Hight[13] observe the spiritual dimension has cognitive, experiential and behavioural aspects. They explain that the cognitive or philosophic aspects include the exploration for meaning, purpose and truth in life. The experiential and emotional aspects include feelings of hope, love, connection, inner peace, comfort and support. They comment that an individual's inner resources, the ability to give and receive spiritual love and the types of relationships with the self, the community, the environment and the transcendent reflect these emotional and experiential aspects. They state that the behavioural aspects of spirituality comprise the way a person 'externally manifests individual spiritual beliefs and the inner spiritual state'.

The 'deeper property of life' to which Hardy refers, is often what resurfaces later. Crisis – illness, bereavement and disappointment – topples barriers, beliefs and defences leaving exposure and naked vulnerability. Jung says every crisis is 'spiritual' in nature – whether it is a conflict in values, a question of life's meaning or purpose or an impasse to the higher self.[14] According to Jung[15] it is when a person reaches the mid-life crisis, just after the 'noon' of life that spiritual values grow and become dominant. Obviously, depending on the life experiences that one encounters, the mid-life crisis may arrive sooner rather than later.

Jung argues that we do not realise the extent to which rationalism, which has destroyed our ability to respond to supernatural symbols and ideas, has put us at the mercy of the psychic underworld. We live in the illusion that we are liberated from superstition, but we have lost our spiritual values to a deeply dangerous degree and the capacity to practise introspection.[16]

This could all seem quite philosophical and abstract but it is relevant to our patients and to us. Postmodern man is passing through a crisis that is existential. Often our lifestyle does not allow us to ask deeper questions about the meaning of our existence. At times, these questions do not arise until some calamity befalls us and we are left defenceless. The diagnoses of angina, congestive cardiac failure, multiple sclerosis or cancer are not simply the findings on an X-ray or MRI scan. The diagnosis falls on someone who has to try to digest it, derive some form of meaning from it and incorporate it into his life philosophy. At times illness – and it does not need to be serious – is the first glimpse we have of our mortality and we do not always like what we see.

General practice prides itself on practising holistic medicine. For example, we need to see a patient with a chronic lung condition in the context of his family and his main carers, his occupation, his environment, the social effects of his illness, his interaction with others and the impact of the condition on his mental and emotional health. However, there is another dimension of health that has remained ignored – at least until recent years – and that is the spiritual dimension.

From a review of the literature on spirituality and health, Pandya[17] found that in the West 87% of the population say that religion and spirituality is an important part of their lives. The *Journal of Family Practice* published a study[18] that showed the beliefs and attitudes of hospital inpatients about faith and prayer and again a survey[19] of the attitudes of physicians and patients to religion. These studies have shown that 77% of patients would like spiritual issues considered as part of their medical care, yet they found that only 10% to 20% of physicians discuss these issues with their patients. As a result, in the USA an increasing number of medical schools offer courses on spirituality and medicine in the medical curriculum.

However, there is a certain taboo about speaking of anything spiritual among many health professionals. It provokes an embarrassed cough, a pregnant silence, a quick change of subject or the pretence that you did not really hear what was being said. It is true that the USA is very different from Britain and people there are more upfront about talking about such matters. In the UK, doctors rarely discuss religion with their patients while 17% of physicians do in the USA. Although the UK is not the USA, this does not alter the fact that the spiritual dimension is an important element for patients in the UK too.

The NHS patients' charter does acknowledge the rights of service users to have their spiritual needs recognised and addressed while the NICE guidelines on cancer services recognises spiritual support for these patients. Yet the spiritual dimension is not just the domain of the terminally ill. Anyone who becomes ill or who faces disruption in his life can find himself in a crisis that is spiritual. He finds himself questioning the meaning and purpose of his existence. He may not know how to articulate this or even be fully conscious that he is doing so. Therefore, the challenge for the health professional is to be aware and alert.

Literature is just one of the many rich sources illustrating the spiritual dimension of patients. Natasha Rostov in Tolstoy's *War and Peace* is such an example. She is engaged to Prince Andrei and falls passionately in love with Anatole – a reckless rake. She is just about to elope with him but, foiled in the attempt, she is brought home shamed and very much a laughing stock in the eyes of St Petersburg society. Above all, she returns nursing a broken heart. Tolstoy continues:

> Natasha's illness was so serious that, fortunately for her and for her parents, the consideration of all that had caused the illness, her conduct and the breaking off of her engagement, receded into the background. She was so ill that it was impossible for them to consider in how far she was to blame for what had happened. She could not eat or sleep, grew visibly thinner, coughed, and, as the doctors made them feel, was in danger. They could not think of anything but how to help her. Doctors came to see her singly and in consultation, talked much in French, German, and Latin, blamed one another, and prescribed a great variety of medicines for all the diseases known to them, but the simple idea never occurred to any of them that they could not know the disease Natasha was suffering from, as no disease suffered by a live man can be known, for every living person has his own peculiarities and always has his own peculiar, personal, novel, complicated disease, unknown to medicine – not a disease of the lungs, liver, skin, heart, nerves, and so on mentioned in medical books, but a disease consisting of one of the innumerable combinations of the maladies of those organs. This simple thought could not occur to the doctors (as it cannot occur to a wizard that he is unable to work his charms) because the business of their lives was to cure, and they

received money for it and had spent the best years of their lives on that business...Natasha's grief began to be overlaid by the impressions of daily life, it
ceased to press so painfully on her heart, it gradually faded into the past, and she
began to recover physically.[20]

It is a clever piece, displaying Tolstoy's perception and knowledge of the actors
who appear on the stage of life: patients, carers and doctors. The doctors fall
into the trap that we fall into every day and that we unwittingly set for ourselves
when we refuse to look at all the dimensions of our patients' health.

The chapters that follow will consider the meaning of holistic healthcare
and search for evidence of our spiritual dimension. We will explore the spiritual
dimension of health through the stories of patients both fictional and non-
fictional. We will attempt to discern the signs that may indicate that a patient is
spiritually distressed and discuss methods of taking a spiritual history. We will
reflect on implications for the health professional. The book concludes with
extracts from the writings of Chiara M conveying her spiritual journey through
a chronic, painful illness.

REFERENCES

1 www.bbc.co.uk/health
2 National Health and Medical Research Council. Promoting the health of the Indigenous Australians. A review of infrastructure support for Aboriginal and Torres Strait
Islander health advancement. Final report and recommendations. Canberra:
NHMRC; 1996. Part 2:4.
3 Bircher J. Towards a dynamic definition of health and disease. *Med Health Care Philos.*
2005; **8**: 335–41.
4 Cottrell RR, Girvan JT, McKenzie JF. *Principles and Foundations of Health Promotion and
Education.* 2nd ed. San Francisco: Benjamin Cummings; 2002.
5 Butler J. *Principles of Health Education and Health Promotion.* 3rd ed. Belmont:
Wadsworth; 2001.
6 Hawks S. Spiritual wellness, holistic health and the practice of health education. *Am
J Health Educ.* 2004; **35**(1): 11–16.
7 Chuengsatiansujp K. Spirituality and health: an initial proposal to incorporate spiritual health in health impact assessment. www.who.int/hia/examples/overview/
whohia203/en/print.html
8 Puchalski CM, Larson DB. Developing curricula in spirituality and medicine. *Acad
Med.* 1998; **73**: 970–4.
9 Gabriel B. Is spirituality good medicine? Bridging the divide between science and
faith. *AAMC Reporter.* 2000; **9**(13): 7–9.
10 Sloan RP, Bagiella E. Spirituality and medical practice: a look at the evidence. *Am Fam
Physician.* 2001; **63**(1): 33–4.
11 Sloan RP, Bagiella E, Powell T. Religion, spirituality, and medicine. *Lancet.* 1999; **353**
(9153): 664–7. Review.

12 Hardy, Sir A. *The Spiritual Nature of Man*. Oxford: Oxford University Press; 1979.
13 Anandarajah G, Hight E. Spirituality and medical practice: using the HOPE questions as a practical tool for spiritual assessment. *Am Fam Physician*. 2001; **63**(1): 81.
14 Seaward BL. Reflections on human spirituality for the worksite. *AJHP*. 1995; 9(3): 165–8.
15 Donatelle RJ, Davis LG. *Access to Health*. 4th ed. Boston: Allyn & Bacon; 1996.
16 Jung CG, Sabini M. *The Earth Has a Soul: CG Jung's Writings on Nature, Technology and Modern Life*. Berkeley: North Atlantic Books; 2002.
17 Pandya L. Spirituality, religion and health. *Geriatric Medicine*. May 2005; 19–22.
18 King DE, Bushwick B. Beliefs and attitudes of hospital inpatients about faith, healing and prayer. *J Fam Pract*. 1994; **39**: 349–52.
19 Maugans TA, Wadland WC. Religion and family medicine: a survey of physicians and patients. *J Fam Pract*. 1991; **32**: 210–13.
20 Tolstoy L. *War and Peace*. 1869. Maude A, Maude L, translators. 1923.

CHAPTER 1

Holistic view of health and illness

'All religions, arts and sciences are branches of the same tree.'
Albert Einstein

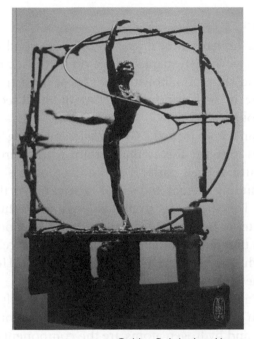

Golden Rule by Lau Hung

One day a home visit to Molly struck me so much that her image remained photographed in my mind. She was elderly and had the gnarled, lumpy fingers of a rheumatoid arthritis sufferer. She had been in incapacitating, chronic intractable pain for several years and all the therapy that she had tried had offered little in the way of relief. Despite this, Molly was optimistic and remained 'healthier' in her outlook than several other people considered objectively to be in 'better health'. She seemed to have an inner resource linked in some way to her health – something of a spiritual nature. Molly and many patients like her are the reason for this book.

HOLISTIC VIEW OF HEALTH

This book is all about 'soul matters' – the spiritual dimension of health. However, to understand the nature and importance of spiritual health, we have to see it in the context of holistic health. This chapter examines the limitations of adopting solely a biomechanical approach towards patients. It examines what we mean by 'holistic health' and it questions why patients often feel unheeded and powerless when they seek medical attention. It argues that to be advocates of holistic practice, we have to consider all the dimensions of health – including the spiritual. This approach reflects WHO's definition of health as 'a state of complete physical, mental and social well-being and not merely the absence of disease or infirmity'.[1]

Meaning of holism

Everyone is talking 'holistic' these days. Not only can you have holistic healthcare, but you can have 'holistic dentistry', go on a 'holistic holiday', have 'holistic education' and shop at a 'holistic bakery' or 'holistic pet supplier'. It is certainly one of the 'in' words and whatever we do, it all seems to be kosher as long as we do it holistically.

The word holism comes from the Greek *'holos'* meaning 'whole'. The Oxford dictionary[2] defines it as 'the theory that certain wholes are to be regarded as greater than the sum of their parts'. It also adds that it is 'the treating of the whole person including mental and social factors rather than just the symptoms of a disease'. The South African philosopher and politician Jan Christian Smuts coined the term 'holism'. He introduced it in his book, *Holism and Evolution*.[3] Smuts sees that matter and life consists of atoms, cells and units which produce natural wholes that we call bodies or organisms. He observes that this feature of 'wholeness' is characteristic of the universe.

Two particular atoms illustrate the idea of holism nicely. A water molecule is much more than the sum of its parts – two hydrogen atoms and one oxygen atom. The oxygen and hydrogen atoms are the components of invisible gases. Oxygen is colourless, tasteless and odourless but we could not live without it. Hydrogen is also imperceptible. Together the two gases combine to form water: a vital, visible liquid, something more much more than the individual constituents. Water quenches thirst, is the gardener's dream when its advent is timely and brings joy and laughter in the swimming pool. Culturally and mythologically over the ages it has been and still is the symbol to many of expiation and purification. Water is also therapeutic and Napoleon Bonaparte once said, 'Water, air, and cleanness are the chief articles in my pharmacy.'

We are 60% water yet I would object if someone were to say that I just consist of water, proteins, carbohydrates, nucleic acids, lipids and vitamins. Being simply defined as a collection of systems for digesting, breathing, thinking, moving and feeling would not fully satisfy me either. There are the physical parts of me, which are to some extent measurable. I am all of these things and much more. I think the term 'holism' embraces the 'much more'. There are the intellectual, emotional, social, cultural and spiritual sides of me. They probably say more about me than all the objectively measurable bits. I am 'much more' than my separate parts.

Consequently, health and illness do not just involve my physical parts but also *me*. Illness will happen to me within my social and cultural context. It therefore follows that adopting a holistic approach to the patient will take account of him as a whole person – body, mind and spirit – rather than just of his symptoms.

To understand the contribution that holism can give to the way we look at health and illness, it might be helpful to look at its opposite – 'reductionism'. Reductionism is the 'doctrine that a system can be fully understood in terms of its isolated parts'.[2] It is based on the mathematical theory promoted by Isaac Newton, the philosophy divulged by René Descartes and the methodology advocated by Francis Bacon.[4] Descartes (1596–1650) viewed the human person as having two distinct and separate realities – the mind and the body. For Descartes the human body was mechanical and worked like a clock. Descartes however left a huge problem that people still debate today: the problem of how the mind works and the link between the mind and the body. Over three and a half centuries later, Descartes' influence still endures in the Western world. Western medicine, modelled on Newtonian mechanics, emphasises the single cause and germ theory of disease. Almost seventy years ago, the coming of antibiotics underlined this further. Gone were the days of purging and leeching. With the case for the single cause and germ theory of disease thus strengthened, the hope arose – understandably – that a pill would be found for every ill. This hope persists today and the pharmaceutical industry produces a wide armamentarium of drugs varying from those used to relieve menopausal symptoms to life-saving drugs to control irregular heart rates and revive the 'dead'. Reductionism has metaphorically and literally been instrumental in working wonders in medicine.

However, the single cause theory does not explain phenomena such as the patient's self-healing ability and that many symptoms result from the body's attempts to right itself. Nonetheless the reductionist world-view permeates the Western understanding of disease and illness in medical literature. It permeates some elements of the media. Headline grabbers such as *'CHOLESTEROL DRUGS SAVE THOUSANDS OF LIVES A YEAR'* or *'DRUG FIRMS RACE AGAINST TIME TO DEVELOP MIRACLE CURE FOR DIABETES'* are examples. The reductionist world-view has led to the widespread prescription of statins to prevent disease when cholesterol levels are normal and drugs to treat hypertension where previously symptomless patients complain bitterly of side effects. The goalposts are constantly changing depending on which study is in vogue. The result? People are left feeling utterly confused leading to a degree of scepticism whenever the next 'health bulletin' is issued. Is chocolate good for you or does it help depression? Should I be drinking a glass of red wine to protect my heart or should I not have any alcohol? Should I be giving my pet Prozac for its depression or should I ask myself when I last took it out for a walk? The contradictions and dilemmas generated by being reductionist are endless.

This story, which I found in a psychiatry book, although rather extreme, is nevertheless telling. Three Martian scientists were sent to earth to discover what makes 'metallic vehicles' (alias cars) speed across the planet. The Martian with the ecologist background discovers the vehicles move at different speeds according to the straightness of the paths and the presence of inexplicable phenomena (alias speed cameras) called 'radar traps'. The second Martian – a psychologist – argues instead that the speed is determined by the age, gender, mood of the individual. The third Martian disagrees and explains speed as a direct result of the chemical process (involving oxygen, fuel and heat) occurring inside an internal-combustion engine. In their own way, each of the Martians is right but singly they do not give the complete picture. This shows the 'potential fallacy of blind reductionism'.[5]

In modern medicine, we fall very much into this blind trap. Much of medical research is driven by reductionism and the 'gold standard' is the randomised controlled trial (RCT). There is the danger that we can hold on to it tenaciously as if it were a cast iron belief system. The front page of a past edition of the *British Medical Journal* (*BMJ*)[6] on evidence based medicine (EBM) encapsulates this. There are three high priests one of which bears a huge tome entitled 'Evidence', while another pours liquid from a bottle called 'Angina' into a boiling cauldron. The third figure tips other items into the cauldron: a stethoscope, pills, 'Rx' and 'Dx' (symbols for treatment and diagnosis). Evidence based medicine does have its limitations because the randomised controlled trial is not suitable for every circumstance, nor is it always the appropriate method to answer our questions. Cohort and case-report studies do not feature highly on the hierarchy of evidence based medicine, yet they often tell us more about the causes and prognosis of illness.

There are champions against the stranglehold of evidence based medicine. The CRAP (Clinicians for the Restoration of Autonomous Practice) Writing Group published a report outlining exactly what its members think about the 'ugly truth' of evidence based medicine.[7] The publication was anonymous to protect the authors from the retaliation of the 'grand inquisitors of the new religion of Evidence Based Medicine'. They claimed the ten commandments of

EBM, presented against a musical background ('All you need is trials') included among its tenets, 'Thou shalt neither publish case reports... and punish those who blaspheme by uttering personal experiences'. The commandments also 'banish unbelievers who partake in qualitative research,' put heathen basic scientists to the rack unless they repent and promise henceforth to randomise all mice, materials and molecules in their experiments. However, CRAP plans to take EBM to court in the Hague for crimes against humanity, challenging the proponents of EBM to provide proof, based on a mega-RCT or a meta-analysis of RCTs that EBM does more good than harm.[7]

A further criticism of evidence based medicine is a potential negative effect on the doctor-patient relationship because of too much emphasis on the rational and quantitative aspects of clinical problems. Human beings are more complex than mechanical objects and their care calls for a more sophisticated, holistic approach. I remember a colleague of mine saying that she would only practise evidence based medicine. While part of me thought that this was laudable the other part recoiled. Medicine is not just about giving patients what 'evidence' suggests. It is not a licence for treating people irresponsibly either.

I was struck by an article of Dr Des Spence.[8] He launches a vitriolic attack against 'lying evidence based medicine' – something which he had previously championed – pointing out that evidence based medicine is not fact but rather a model to interpret available evidence. He states that ten years in general practice gives a complete longitudinal knowledge of disease and people that no study will ever able to convey: 'knowledge, even evidence based knowledge, I have come to realise, is no substitute for life experience'.[8]

MOVING BEYOND THE BIOMEDICAL MODEL
The many dimensions of health and illness
A holistic perspective of health and illness takes in the physical, emotional, social, cultural, psychological and spiritual dimensions of the person. The physical dimension is the most obvious. It is 'matter' and measurable and therefore the one that doctors most underline when it comes to collecting symptoms. How important are all the other dimensions? Does considering them make any difference to patient care?

Social dimension
The social dimensions of health and illness have been known since Hippocrates. He was a strict observer not just of clinical symptoms but of the customs of different peoples, their environments and the effects these had had on their health. For Hippocrates the good physician had to

This model, based on the biopsychosocial model of illness, illustrates where the spiritual dimension might be incorporated. Sometimes the spiritual dimension may be the most important aspect of the illness:

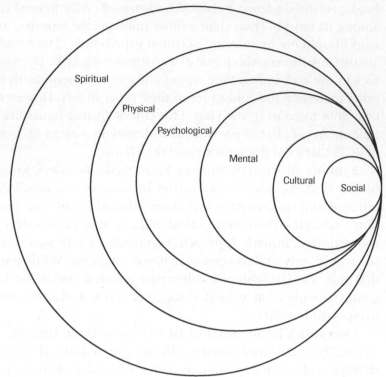

Sometimes other dimensions of an illness may be more important as in these examples. Here the physical dimension is the most important aspect of the illness:

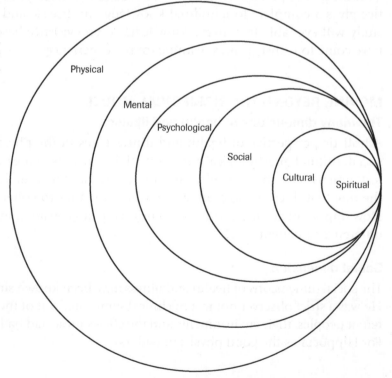

Here the
psychological
dimension of the
illness is the most
important:

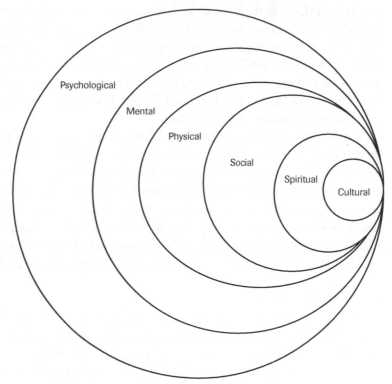

FIGURE 1.1 Dimensions of health and of illness.

> ...consider the waters which the inhabitants use, whether they be marshy and soft,
> or hard, and running from elevated and rocky situations, and then if saltish and unfit
> for cooking...the mode in which the inhabitants live, and what are their pursuits,
> whether they are fond of drinking and eating to excess, and given to indolence, or
> are fond of exercise and labour, and not given to excess in eating and drinking.[9]

Social deprivation and poverty affect health. Dickens wrote graphically of this.
One of his most pitiable characters is Jo, the orphan in *Bleak House* who skulks
in Tom-all-Alone's:

> Jo lives – that is to say, Jo has not yet died – in a ruinous place, known to the like
> of him by the name of Tom-all-Alone's...so these ruined shelters have bred a
> crowd of foul existence that crawls in and out of gaps in walls and boards...where
> the rain drips in; and comes and goes fetching and carrying fever.[10]

Poor Jo eventually dies in his childhood.

Parents have asked me many times if the dampness in the walls of their
council house is contributing to 'Jimmy's asthma'. They have asked for a letter

to support them in their bid to be rehoused because of the 'mould on the walls'. Initially there was not much 'evidence' from studies to suggest that this was the case and yet the parents' assertions seemed to make sense. It therefore comes as no surprise that a 2007 study showed that improving the indoor environment may lead to improved self-rated health, fewer visits to a general practitioner, fewer days off work and off school.[11] Poor housing is usually associated with poverty, poor health and social ills.

At the end of 2006, the *BMJ*[12] conducted a poll asking its readership to vote which they considered the greatest milestone in medical history during the last 166 years. The competition was stiff: from Louis Pasteur's germ theory in 1862 to Crick and Watson's paper proposing the double helix structure of DNA. The greatest innovation in medicine was not voted to be the antibiotic, or anaesthetic or the discovery of X-rays but the introduction of clean water and an efficient sewage system. The irony is the champion behind the 'sanitary revolution' was not a medical doctor or a sanitary engineer but a lawyer and social reformer.

Cultural dimension

Culture and the meaning we give to illness and health are closely bound. Illness is synonymous with sickness, disease, affliction, disability; while health equates with haleness, robustness, vigour, well-being and strength. Culture relates to the customs, achievements and civilisation of a particular people so of course it has implications for health and illness.

Our medical textbooks abound with definitions of all sorts of disease – chronic obstructive pulmonary disease, coronary artery disease and chronic liver disease etc. Doctors see disease as an objectively verified disorder of bodily functions or systems associated with an identifiable group of signs and symptoms. For example, doctors know that chronic obstructive pulmonary disease (normally translated as 'chronic bronchitis') is a common progressive disorder of airway obstruction with little or no reversibility (meaning 'inhalers don't always work').[13] Illness instead is the patient's subjective experience. Locker describes illness as a social phenomenon consisting of the 'meaning actors employ to make sense of observed or experienced events'.[14] It is dependent 'not solely on biological mechanisms, no matter how crucial they are, but on convergences between biology and culture'.[15]

I love Jane Austen. She is witty, perceptive, perspicacious *and* she has an accurate knowledge of human nature. She could be writing about people today minus parasols, muslin gowns, eyeglasses and tailcoats. Lady Bertram in *Mansfield Park* suffers from laziness, which she labels as ill health. She exhibits perfect illness behaviour that is culturally acceptable as she lies 'sunk back in one corner of the sofa, the picture of health, wealth, ease, and tranquillity'.[16] Anne Elliot's sister, Mary, in *Persuasion* similarly lounges on a sofa. She is 'often a little unwell, and always thinking a great deal of her own complaints, and always in the habit of claiming Anne when anything was the matter'. Mary comments, 'I am so ill I can hardly speak. I have not seen a creature the whole morning!' While her husband, Charles Musgrove, confidentially whispers into one of Anne's ears: 'I wish you could persuade Mary not to be always fancying herself ill.' Mary declares into the other: 'I do believe if Charles were to see me dying, he would not think there was anything the matter with me. I am sure, Anne, if you would, you might persuade him that I really am very ill – a great deal worse than I ever own.' However, Mary rallies and becomes completely well whenever life departs from the mundane in the form of a walk, pleasant society, a ball. Mary and Lady Bertram label their problems in coping with life as illness. They both share an equal measure of indolence.[17]

Illness involves the departure from a state considered normal or routine. This 'departure' is expressed in various ways. There may be a change in physical structure or appearance such as the crippling effects of arthritis. There may be the change in subjective experience such as the lancinating pain of a cluster headache or trigeminal neuralgia. There may be a change in activity, mood or behaviour as in the apathetic, saddened state of depression. There may be certain behaviour associated with an underlying disorder – behaviour such as staying in bed, not going out, doing little physical activity. This illness behaviour may seem to be culturally appropriate or inappropriate: lying in bed for 10 days with a cut finger would universally be considered bizarre.

Transcultural researchers in psychiatry have criticised the West for incorporating depression, regarded as a Western construct, into the international classification of diseases.[18] For example, the reaction to bereavement varies in different cultures. In the West, there may be what we describe as the classic picture of depression with apathy, hopelessness and low mood. However, Sri Lankan Buddhists cope with the loss of a loved one by meditating on the illusory nature of the world and its pleasures. The Kaluli of New Guinea respond to bereavement with anger and the expectation of compensation from society for the bereaved individual. Iranian children see their loss in a historical context – the suffering of their martyrs. These coping measures have been referred to as a 'work of culture'.[18] Ignorance of another's culture could lead to labels of 'abnormality' if not disease. They could also result in inappropriate therapy and medicalisation.

Within a population, culture may vary with time. The picture of health in Edwardian times was of a plump, rosy, well-endowed woman. This is an anathema today in the West and for some the 'ideal' woman is the skinny, size zero nymph sporting Gucci attire. Instead, others would even define such models as sufferers of chronic malnutrition.

Psychological and emotional dimensions of illness

I can recall many stories: patients whose cancer began after intense anxiety; patients who began to suffer from destructive arthritis after a protracted period of stress; patients whose multiple sclerosis began following severe mental or emotional trauma. I am sure that if asked people will relate the onset of their illness to a specific life event – bereavement, a disappointment, a divorce, a redundancy. Recent bereavement and relocation of the elderly are considered to be associated with increased morbidity and mortality from a wide range of disorders.[19] No one can adequately explain the reasons for this increase in illness, but possibilities include the loss of care and companionship, personal neglect and stress induced neuroendocrine changes. Occasionally people take ill or consult their doctor at or around the time of an anniversary of the death of a loved one or other major loss.

How many heroines become seriously ill or even die of a broken heart after some disappointment! There is Caroline Helstone in Charlotte Bronte's *Shirley*[20] who pines and physically ails for the love of Robert Moore and Marianne who almost dies following the perfidy of Willoughby in *Sense and Sensibility*.[21]

The idea of stress inducing changes in the endocrine and immunology systems has existed for several years. It is called psychoneuroimmunology and involves many disciplines – psychiatry, psychology, neurology, internal medicine, endocrinology and immunology being some examples. It is concerned with interactions between the brain (mind/behaviour) and the immune system and the clinical effects produced. Robert Ader first coined the term in the 1970s. The field has grown so much in recent decades that at the time of writing, a major tome by Ader with over thirteen hundred pages on the subject has reached its fourth edition.[22]

A landmark paper published by Ader and Cohen more than thirty years ago established the importance of communication between the brain and the immune system.[23] They managed to prolong the life of mice with an autoimmune disease by using saccharin as a conditioned stimulus to produce the immunosuppression properties of cyclophosphamide – a drug used to treat autoimmune disease. Studies on humans have looked at psychological stress and the common cold. In one study, 276 volunteers were inoculated with a common cold virus and then checked to see if they developed the condition. The presence of severe chronic stress for more than a month was found to be linked to a substantial increase in the risk of the disease.[24]

In another study[25] over 300 healthy volunteers were given nasal drops containing a common cold virus. The researchers found that volunteers who had positive emotions such as a greater tendency to be happy, pleased and relaxed were less likely to suffer from the cold virus compared with the volunteers who had a greater tendency to experience negative emotions such as anxiety, hostility and depression. A further study involving 2000 middle-aged men followed-up over a 20-year period showed that depression was associated with an increased risk of the occurrence of and death from cancer.[26]

The research in psychoneuroimmunology is intriguing and far beyond the scope of this book. It raises more questions than it answers. Cytokines are soluble messenger molecules that determine much of the immune system's ability to communicate between different comportments. Once cytokines reach their destination cells they produce varying effects depending on the type of cytokines and the cells that they target. Generally, cytokines will send signals that activate or divide certain cells. They may direct specific cells to particular areas of the body. Studies have shown that cytokines producing inflammation can be the result of negative emotions and stressful experiences.

Psychoneuroimmunology may provide a foundation for understanding the biological basis of humanistic medicine and of alternative or complementary medical techniques. It offers the hope of developing new non-linear models of health and disease. However over 2000 years ago, Aristotle said:

> Psyche and body react sympathetically to each other, it seems to me. A change in the state of the psyche produces a change in the structure of the body, and conversely, a change in the structure of the body produces a change in the state of the psyche.

Somewhat nearer our own time, Sir Francis Bacon similarly suggested:

> Let us enquire how and how far the humours and affects of the body do alter and work upon the mind, or again, how and how far the passions or apprehensions of the mind do alter or work on the body.

Did these wise men understand something that we appear to have lost and stand in need of recovering?

MEANING OF ILLNESS

Pietroni[27] speaks of six different modes or languages to assign a meaning to illness. They are:

1 medical/material/molecular
2 psychological/psychosomatic/psychoanalytical
3 preventive/promotional/anticipatory
4 cultural/social/political
5 archetypal/metaphorical/symbolic
6 space/time/energy.

The medical/material/molecular mode is the language of classical science and is epitomised by a mechanistic representation of the body. The words of Descartes, 'I think of the human body as a machine' are as celebrated as Humphrey Bogart's misquoted, 'Play it again, Sam.' Using the Descartes model, doctors look for the cause of illness and set out on a quest of eradication, extermination and elimination. This type of model leaves many questions unanswered and patients and often doctors feel that it does not provide us with the whole story.

The psychological/psychosomatic/psychoanalytical mode helps the patient uncover the underlying reason for the illness. The idea is that addressing the underlying cause of the illness is important for its treatment. Many have contributed to this field – Michael Balint[28] among them. He was a psychoanalyst who practiced in London after the war. He began a discussion and support group for family doctors, gaining tremendous insight into the machinations of the consultation. His work provided many useful concepts for our understanding of the doctor-patient relationship, including the idea of the doctor being the 'drug' and the dependant 'sick role' which the doctor permits the patient to adopt. I agree that sometimes *I* am the drug. I have had patients tell me that they felt better just talking to me. I interpreted it simply as polite exaggeration until I discovered that sometimes it is actually true.

The preventive/promotional/anticipatory mode is the language of health education. This is very popular in the Western world. Strategies vary from measures such as 'traffic light' food labelling to overdosing with high dose vitamins, from successive fads of drinking pomegranate juice to dousing, creaming and bathing with Aloe vera. Aloe vera has become the 'healthy' choice panacea – a symbol of the search to do everything to keep fit and well. It often follows that if people reason like this, when they are unwell they will ask if something is missing from the diet and if taking many supplements would help. Thus, the preventive, promotional mode can just end up being a narrow form of reductionism, a guilt trip where every ill is attributed to a 'lack' of something.

The cultural/social/political mode involves the cultural and social attitudes of patients and health professionals and their impact on the meaning of illness. I have touched on this to some extent already.

The archetypal/metaphorical/symbolic mode seeks for the meaning of illness in folklore, myths and legends. It searches for the meaning of illness in the arts. In archetypal medicine, illness brings people together in groups (e.g. patient groups) and addresses the need for a collective experience.

The sixth mode consists of space/time/energy and here the human body is seen as a bioenergetic organism – an empty space within an even greater empty space. I find it daunting to think that reducing the space between all the electrons and nuclei in all the atoms found in a single human body would result in our being no more than the size of a grain of sand. It brings to mind the Old Testament saying about Abraham's descendants being as a many as the grains of sand on the seashore. The space/time/energy mode regards illness as the result of a disturbance of collective field forces – hence the interest in some of the complementary therapies that consider themselves 'energy medicine'. Therapeutic touch and Reiki therapy are some examples.

We try to understand our experience of illness and we all have our models. Susan Sontag strongly believes that illness should not be described with metaphor and that the most truthful and salutary way of regarding illness is one most purified of and resistant to metaphoric thinking.[29] Madam de Vercellis in Rousseau's *Confessions*[30] does not show the least evidence of metaphoric thinking during her last illness. She demonstrates such fortitude that Rousseau sees her die without showing any weakness or limitation. She continues until her last breath as if dying were the most commonplace thing in the world.

However, for many of us, metaphor characterises our lives. We have used stories from time immemorial to explain our lives and our experiences. It is enough to look at Greek mythology. There are myths like the story of Demeter and her sorrow at the loss of her daughter Persephone to the realm of the underworld. During her three months of sorrow, she forbids 'the trees to yield fruit and the earth to grow'.[31] Persephone's return to the earth brings a welcome spring. There are stories, which our parents have told us on countless occasions, about what happens to naughty girls and boys when they persist in their bad habits. Stories, myths and metaphor are in some way intrinsic to human nature. Similarly, as illness is something that we experience, in an attempt to give it meaning and make it comprehensible, we ultimately end up resorting to metaphor!

Sometimes metaphor is more visible than audible. Oliver Wendell Holmes opened a new building at Harvard Medical School in 1883 with these words: 'I have often wished that disease could be hunted by its professional antagonists in couples – a doctor and a doctor's quick-witted wife.' He goes on to observe that many a suicide would have been prevented because the doctor's wife would have seen in the merchant's face his impending bankruptcy while her 'stupid husband' was prescribing for his dyspepsia. She would have recognised that a maiden was lovelorn by her 'ill-adjusted ribbon' and a droop in the attitude – things that are meaningless to her spouse.[32] To convey, understand, diagnose and treat illness patients and healthcare workers may need to use metaphor.

HOLISTIC HEALTHCARE

A really good liver

I remember scenes from medical school – the excitement of going round the wards with a keen doctor who would take us to feel a 'really good spleen' or make us listen to an 'interesting cardiac murmur'. Like my fellow students in new, pristine white coats, I was very enthusiastic. However, something in me rebelled and a little voice said, 'This isn't quite right.' It was not that we did not greet the patient, ask permission to examine and do all that medical etiquette and politeness required. It is just that I felt uneasy and could not articulate why. One day the professor invited my group to examine a 'really good liver'. We all trotted behind him and assembled around the patient's bedside. I recognised her distinctive face immediately. I thought, 'This isn't a liver – I *know* her!' It is a lesson that remained with me throughout the rest of medical school and my practice of medicine. I had to see patients in their entirety and not as fragmented parts. This entirety is a person.

This is the vision that holistic healthcare promotes. The British Holistic Medical Association (BHMA)[33] believes the core values of compassion, respect, open-mindedness, competence and self-care should underpin holistic practice and that they should be incorporated into the daily lives of practitioners and patients. The General Medical Council shares all of these core values, however in the booklet 'Good Medical Practice'[34] it refers frequently to care but not to compassion. The BHMA goes some steps further as it champions whole person approaches, especially within the NHS. It supports ways to incorporate holism into healthcare organisations and encourages research that seeks a holistic understanding of health and healing.

Each individual is unique and holism underlines this uniqueness. Holism sees people as parts of a family, culture and community and regards people as entities with physical, psychological, sociocultural and spiritual aspects.[35] Some consider that holistic health is based on the law of nature where a whole consists of interdependent parts. The earth is made up of systems such as air, land, water, plants and animals and what happens to one affects the other. Similarly, the individual is also composed of interdependent parts that are physical, mental, emotional and spiritual. When one part is not working fully this has an impact on other parts of the person. How many of us get 'the runs' before an important event – particularly when we have to perform in public? How many poor sufferers are bound to experience a severe attack of migraine on a certain day of the week because it is the most stressful one?

Comparing holistic healthcare with the earth and its systems is applying the idea of holism on an enormous scale. Iain Scott, a passionate lover of wildlife, sees that life is interconnected and that if we destroy or alter an ecosystem, thereby threatening the natural balance of the planet, we threaten some or all of the species within it.[36] He comments that 'interconnectedness is a basic principle of nature' and that unique individual specimens and species exist within a wider interrelated and interdependent ecosystem. He calls for a paradigm shift that makes us look beyond one unit – the self – to the greater whole.

Jeffrey Sachs, an economist, arrives at the same conclusion. Using a term coined by the scientist Paul Crutzen – 'the Anthropocene' (human created era of the Earth's history) – he says that human beings for the first time have taken hold not only of the economy and of population dynamics but also of the planet's physical systems. However, he considers that ensuring that we continue with human successes 'without going right over the cliff will prove to be our generation's greatest challenge'.[37] Redressing our planet's problems requires a holistic approach, which looks at not only economic development but also poverty alleviation, health and aid policy, and environmental sustainability.

Other voices protest against the short-sightedness of people who fail to recognise the interconnectedness of life and its components. For biologist Mae-Wan Ho,[38] in genetic engineering there is an unholy alliance between bad science and big business that works indefatigably for one self-interested aim: profit. A scientist with much experience in genetics, she argues that modern, reductionist scientific thinking sees the world as bits and pieces without acknowledging the existence of organisms, eco-systems, societies and communities. She believes that genetic engineering poses real risks for humanity with nightmarish scenarios of genes hopping from one species to the other and the creation of super viruses. She thinks that the unnatural techniques used in genetic engineering such as the construction of artificial viruses designed to cross species barriers in an enhanced way promote this. Holistic practice is imperative but not just in ecology and science. We need to increase this practice in medicine.

Advances in medical science have meant an increase in medical technology with powers of diagnosis that would have been the envy of Hippocrates himself. Technology has come with a price. It is a double-edged sword, an unwitting source of division between health professionals and their patients as a doctor, Rafael Campo, describes in his poem 'Technology and Medicine'.[39] He speaks of how he came to see himself and I would venture to say, how patients sometimes see doctors:

> The transformation is complete. My eyes
> Are microscopes and cathode X-ray tubes
> In one, so I can see bacteria,
> Your underwear, and even through to bones.
> My hands are hypodermic needles, touch
> Turned into blood: I need to know your salts
> And chemistries, a kind of intimacy
> That won't bear pondering. It's more than love,
> More weird than ESP...my mouth, for instance,
> So small and sharp, a dry computer chip
> That never gets to kiss or taste or tell
> A brief truth like 'You're beautiful,' or worse,
> 'You're crying just like me; you are alive.'

The void that CAM fills

In the UK and many parts of the world, patients are voting with their feet. In Britain, surveys have shown that as many as 30% of the population has used complementary medicine. Patients express dissatisfaction with the care they receive from their general practitioners and hospital doctors. I have often heard expressions such as 'He didn't *listen* to me,' 'He had written the prescription *before* I had even finished,' 'She didn't *even* examine me!' There is a reluctance to take pharmaceutical drugs and the added perception that they have many, noxious side effects. New medical terms such as 'pharmacovigilance' and 'pharmacoepidemiology' confirm these suspicions. Patients also perceive a lack of holistic care from conventional practitioners.

Studies show various reasons why patients use complementary medicine. Some reasons are:

➤ dissatisfaction with conventional medicine
➤ additional support in chronic illness
➤ the lack of holism in conventional medicine
➤ the perceived greater sense of self-control with complementary medicine.

Such patients feel that a holistic viewpoint is important to their care and that conventional doctors did not necessarily possess this. They also think the state of mind and emotions play an important part in their health and that doctors should give this more attention. They want more comprehensive explanations about illness. They do not merely want a diagnosis.[40]

Despite the many objections raised against complementary medicine – and the main one is the lack of robust 'evidence' (namely the randomised controlled trial to minimise bias) – complementary medicine remains popular. John Diamond, a journalist who died in 2001 of cancer, had no doubts about the inefficaciousness of CAM (Complementary and Alternative Medicine). In his last, unfinished book, he attempts to debunk the myth surrounding CAM[41] and expose its quackery. His is one of many voices. A well-known professor of surgery, observing that homeopathy is closer to witchcraft than science, writes that for him alternative medicines are unproven and based on 'conceptual beliefs of human biology that are ancient, metaphysical and simply wrong.' Those who think otherwise imply a denial of progress in our knowledge of human anatomy, physiology and biology. Like others, he considers that some of the complementary approaches might be in the psychosocial domain and others in the spiritual domain, 'acting as surrogates for religious faith in a secular society'.[42] This may well be a valid argument. Centuries ago, the roles of the priest and doctor were united in one person and that is still the case in some societies. It is enough to think of the shaman.

To counter these arguments, George Lewith, a physician and researcher in complementary medicine argues that the evidence about CAM 'is not a barren wasteland'.[43] A large meta-analysis study reports that the effects of homeopathy cannot be simply dismissed as placebo.[44] A similar study using different methodology concludes that homeopathic medicine has no specific therapeutic effect.[45] Nothing daunted, Lewith says, 'It may be the very specific quality, content and context of the homeopathic consultation that is the key to success, through its ability to empower patients with chronic illness.'[43] He defiantly adds, '…perhaps conventional medicine might learn from this?'

The debate continues. Although there is a lack of scientific evidence proving that complementary medicine works, patients and practitioners attest that it *does* achieve clinical results. Some practitioners prefer to speak of the clinical 'legitimacy' of CAM rather than to dwell on its lack of scientific legitimacy.[46]

It is not all plain sailing with pharmaceutical drugs either. A study showed that 21% of the 160 most commonly prescribed drugs in the USA were given on an off-label basis (that is they were used to treat conditions for which no licence had been granted). The authors concluded that off-label medication is common in outpatient care and that most of it occurs without scientific support.[47] Sleeping tablets are considered neither safe nor effective in the long-term[48] (although some patients might choose to differ in opinion!) and yet they still feature regularly in the top 20 most prescribed drugs in the UK and the USA. Clinical 'legitimacy' features in conventional medicine too.

Doctors – probably much more than other health professionals – remain uncomfortable with the word 'holism'. A doctor reported that he attended a prestigious international conference in Orlando.[49] A series of studies were presented and one examined the extent to which Swedish GPs considered that a holistic approach was important to their work. The presentation of the paper was not eligible for CME (continuing medical education) credits – the conference organisers possibly thinking that 'holism' was about alternative medicine and so something unscientific. The irony is that the study had been motivated by EURACT (the European Academy of Teachers of General Practice),[50] which defines 'holistic modelling' as one of the 'six core competencies of the GP/family doctor'. The organisation states that dealing with health problems in their '-physical, psychological, social, cultural and existential dimensions' is characteristic of general practice.

Charlton also does not like the term 'holism', affirming the ideal kind of doctor is not the holistic one but rather 'the humane doctor should be our ultimate aspiration'.[51] For him 'holistic medicine' lacks precise meaning and he considers there is a special connotation when it is attached to champions of alternative therapies. He condemns the 'moral criticism' of orthodox medicine implicit in the understanding of holistic medicine held by these champions.

There is the belief almost to the point of dogma that complementary means holistic but this is not necessarily the case. There are many examples of CAM that per se do not consider health holistically. After all what is holistic about being cleaned out with a coffee enema, being pricked by acupuncture needles or being prescribed a herbal remedy or homeopathic medicine if the practitioner himself does not adopt a holistic approach?

A 'conventional' or a CAM practitioner may not necessarily ask about a patient's diet and social circumstances, discern that his problem is possibly psychosomatic or that his symptoms started following an existential crisis in his life. However is it important to adopt a holistic perspective of the patient especially in modern general practice and hospital care with their time constraints, the points and rewards driven systems and league tables? What do practitioners themselves think? A survey of almost 4000 GPs in Scotland revealed that nearly 9 in 10 thought that a holistic approach was necessary to provide good healthcare. Only 21% of these GPs felt that primary care was delivering holistic care of a high standard. Seventy-three per cent felt that this lack of a holistic perspective led to higher rates of prescribing, 63% considered that it resulted in more referrals to secondary care and 57% thought that it led to an increased demand for complementary therapies. Sixty-seven per cent agreed that psychological factors played an important role in organic physical disease. Time was one of the constraints to the delivery of holistic care.[52] Whole-person approaches reduce the burden of symptoms and hospital referrals. They also lead to greater patient satisfaction. We may agree to disagree on the definition of holistic health but it is clear that patients do want it and they often feel that their doctors and carers are unable to deliver it.

Complexity science is just another way – I think – of speaking about adopting holistic principles. A complex adaptive system is a group of individual agents with freedom to act in ways that cannot always be determined. These actions are interconnected so the action of one part changes the context of the other agents.[53] Complexity is a scientific theory that claims that some systems display behavioural phenomena that are completely inexplicable by any standard analysis of the systems' constituent parts. These phenomena are commonly referred to as emergent behaviour. They appear to occur in many complex systems involving living organisms, such as the stock market or the human brain.[54] In human health and illness there are several layers of such systems including 'wider social, political and cultural systems which can influence outcomes in entirely novel and unpredictable ways'.[53] Another important observation is that a small change in one part of the network of interacting systems may induce a much larger change in another part through what are known as amplification effects.

How far complexity science is useful in demonstrating the intricacies of human disease is questionable. Nonetheless, if we apply complexity science to medicine, it is logical to conclude that illness cannot be modelled in a simple cause and effect system. The single germ theory is too simplistic a model to adequately explain and treat illness in our patients.

Every condition is psychosomatic

Darian Leader and David Corfield[55] have written a fascinating book, which questions why people get ill. They set off with a whole series of 'whys'. Why are people who are more socially isolated likely to get ill? Why is a sufferer of rheumatoid arthritis more likely to experience a flare-up of her condition if she is facing emotional conflict? Why are asthma sufferers more likely to have better lung functioning if they write about troubling experiences in their lives? They conclude the more an illness is studied within the context of a patient's life as a whole, the less dependable are routine, universally accepted explanations. The book unearths some of the interesting research and case studies buried deep in the bowels of the history of Western medicine since the first half of the last century. Leader and Corfield discover that 'psychosomatic medicine' takes on a new meaning and that any disorder could be approached psychosomatically – from the common cold to malaria.

Past generations of doctors seem to have been much more aware of adopting a whole-person approach. Schlaegel's textbook on psychosomatic ophthalmology[56] was a standard text for the medical profession in the USA. He writes, 'The doctor who neglects the role of emotions robs himself and his patients of the tools for diagnosis and therapy.' He eliminates some of the most powerful agents in the development of disease.

He regards every condition as psychosomatic ('psyche' meaning mind and 'soma' body) because both psychological and somatic factors have a part in its course. For him, psychosomatic ophthalmology is an approach where in an addition to a thorough physical examination, there is a psychological one. The 'mutual interrelation' of the two aspects is then studied together.

Ophthalmologists of the time considered that anything from 40% to 100% of their eye cases involved emotional conflict. Bizarre as it may seem, Schlaegel speaks of Inman, an ophthalmologist who observed that an intense interest in childbirth was an important factor in the development of a chalazion (cyst on eyelid). In over 200 consecutive cases 80% displayed a strong interest in childbirth compared with 23.4% in a control group. An example is a 33-year-old man who had surgery for chalazion (stye) of both eyelids. The left chalazion disappeared but the right one enlarged. He returned three months later for further treatment. Inman then told him that he suspected he had been particularly interested in a baby's birth during the three-month interval. After initially faltering, the patient confided that his sister-in-law had had her first baby.

> When asked why he had been so greatly interested, the patient said that 14 years previously he had undergone an unsuccessful operation for undescended testicles and could never have a child. He did not inform his wife of this until 18 months after their marriage. She had not reproached him, but the patient knew that her sister's pregnancy had stirred his wife's longing for a child.

Schlaegel also suggests that in some cases excessive involuntary lacrimation is due to 'a constant plea to be loved'. One of the cases which illustrates this is a woman who complained of a watery left eye. The tear passages were found to be patent. Further history revealed the episodes of lacrimation occurred at the ages of 22, 43 and 45 – critical moments of actual or threatened separation from her mother.

A proposed framework for holistic care

One of the obstacles to adopting a more holistic approach to medicine is the lack of a workable, usable framework. The integral theory of the contemporary philosopher Ken Wilber[57] might be a good starting point. Specific aspects of Wilber's theory have been applied in areas as diverse as business and marine ecology. Ken Wilber's 4-quadrant model interfaces exterior and interior dimensions with those of the individual and collective.

Table 1.1 Astin's adaptation of Wilber's 4-quadrant model.[57]

Upper Left: 'I' *Interior-Individual*	*Upper Right: 'It'* *Exterior-Individual*
Feelings	Organs
Meanings	Tissues
Concepts	Cells
Beliefs	Behaviour
Lower Left: 'We' *Interior-Collective*	*Lower Right: 'Its'* *Exterior-Collective*
Shared meanings	Social structures
Cultural beliefs	Families, tribes
Shared world-views	Ecosystems
Value subcultures	Communities

We could apply Wilber's theory to Len's case. Len, an elderly gentleman, comes to the consulting room accompanied by a family friend who is concerned about his behaviour. Len has decided to step down from the family business and to divide it among his daughters according to their profession of love. The friend, Earl Kent, describes how 'the dotage of old age had so clouded over his reason' that he could no longer discern 'truth from flattery, nor a gay painted speech from words that came from the heart'. His friend goes on to describe other features about Len, which reveal profound change. There is clearly a loss of his intellectual and cognitive functions. A few questions reveal that Len probably has senile dementia – the correct diagnosis. This is the 'exterior-individual' aspect of Len. There is a possibility that Len might benefit from Aricept, the dementia drug, and as a doctor you note that, although he does not live with any close family members, his friend appears supportive. End of consultation.

However, this is only one dimension of Len's life and it certainly does not reveal the full extent of his tragic story. To do this we would have to explore his feelings, the meaning he attributes to his experiences and his belief system (interior-individual). The family friend gives more history. He says that when anyone challenged Len about his unjust behaviour in sharing out his youngest daughter's inheritance with the other two, he became irrationally angry. 'Like a frantic patient who kills his physician and loves his mortal disease', he threatened his friend with death if he ever saw him again. In his mental state Len believes that his youngest daughter has wronged him. Her plain, honest speech is for him a demonstration of a lack of love. He acts according to his altered belief system and his idea of what is right and wrong.

Len's illness however takes place within a shared culture (the interior-we). The 'exterior-its' are Len's family, his employers, his business empire and the entire social structure around him. There is a shared cultural idea of how Len – the former owner of the business – should be treated. Respect is due to him. However, Len has behaved like a fool and he ends up being treated as such by his daughters and even by former employers. One of his favourite employees describes the situation well:

> And I for sorrow sung,
> That such a king should play bo-peep,
> And go the fools among.[58]

Len's degradation reaches its lowest point when he manages to escape from a place of safety and is found wandering about the fields

> in a pitiable condition, stark mad, and singing aloud to himself with a crown upon his head which he had made of straw, and nettles, and other wild weeds that he had picked up in the cornfields.[59]

Isolating Len's symptoms from the whole drama that is going on around him would not do justice to his case. A practitioner would fail to understand the depth of his suffering and how best to help him.

All the systems fail here: Len's mind and body; his family; his social fabric; his 'kingdom'. This parody of Shakespeare's *King Lear* is of course an extreme example but the challenge for health professionals is to place each patient within the context of his story with all the social, cultural, psychological and spiritual dimensions. So often we stop at Len, without filming him 'in location' with his kingship and kingdom.

Marianne in *Sense and Sensibility*[21] is another example of the importance of looking at our patients holistically and piecing together their stories. She illustrates all the dimensions of health/illness. Marianne had an 'excess of sensibility' and following a disappointment at the beginning of Jane Austen's book, she and her mother encouraged each other…in the violence of their affliction. The agony of grief which overpowered them at first was voluntarily renewed, was sought for, was created again and again. They gave themselves up wholly to their sorrow, seeking increase of wretchedness in every reflection that could afford it, and resolved against ever admitting consolation in the future.

This description of Marianne's character is a presage of what is to come later in the story when Willoughby jilts her. Through neglecting her health, she becomes very ill and reaches the point of death. In one of the closing chapters of the book, she comments that her illness has made her think and given her leisure and calmness for serious recollection: 'I saw that my own feelings had prepared my sufferings, and that my want of fortitude under them had almost led me to the grave.'

Holism in its truest essence is not solely associated with 'conventional' or 'complementary' medicine. Each of the proponents of these fields can be reductionist to the extreme. Holistic healthcare embraces the physical, psychological, mental, emotional, social and spiritual dimensions. In a given patient in a given time one or more of these dimensions may be more predominant, even though they are unavoidably linked to each other.

Pietroni describes a case of a 27-year-old Spanish man presenting with the classic symptoms and signs of a duodenal ulcer subsequently proven by investigation.[27] He had left his native country after an affair with his colleague's wife and found himself unsettled and unemployed in London. He was a practising Christian and much troubled by the relationship. Eating sporadically and drinking heavily, he had noticed a growing inability to sit still and incapacity to concentrate for any length of time. The practitioner treats the patient according to the meaning that he – the therapist – gives to the illness and the model that he uses.

According to Pietroni's[27] previously mentioned model, the practitioner focussing on the medical/material mode will decide the cause of the illness is overproduction of acid in the stomach and prescribe a drug that reduces acid production. The practitioner who highlights the psychological dimension of the case might explore issues concerning the extramarital affair. A third practitioner might highlight the need to alter the diet, reduce alcohol and make other necessary lifestyle changes. The fourth practitioner might consider the problem is sociocultural. He may direct his attention towards helping the patient to have suitable housing and employment. A fifth practitioner might see the illness as a manifestation of the patient's underlying feelings of remorse and his guilt-ridden conscience. After all, a dictionary definition of an ulcer is a 'moral blemish', 'a corroding or corrupting influence'.[2] The sixth practitioner may consider, like Einstein, that field is the only reality and see the human individual as a bioenergetic organism – an empty space in an even emptier space.

In this space/time/energy paradigm, he may view illness as a result of an upset in the collective field force and decide to use methods such as meditation and group activity.

A practitioner with a holistic approach might consider all of these dimensions – perhaps weighing up the relative importance of each in a particular case. Together they make up the physical, psychological, social, cultural, spiritual and mental dimensions of the patient. It is true that giving the patient an anti-ulcer drug prescription might settle his symptoms, but if his symptoms keep returning...

To conclude, it is limiting to look at any phenomenon (a patient's illness, a natural disaster, global warming, a fall in business profits) with just one lens. An Indian fable, shows the short-sightedness of such an approach. Six men – blind from birth – wanted to know the shape and form of an elephant. They individually approached it from a different angle. They then got together to describe how each one envisaged the elephant. The first said that it was like a great mud wall, hard-baked in the hot sun. The second believed that it had the shape of a spear. The third thought that it was like a rope. The fourth said that it was like a serpent while the fifth like a fan. The sixth declared it was like the trunk of a great palm tree. Each in his own little way was right, but each was also wrong.

We have touched on the cultural, social and psychological dimensions of illness in this chapter. The next chapter looks at the meaning of the 'spiritual dimension'. 'Spiritual' is another word with which many feel uncomfortable. 'Unscientific', 'nothing to do with medicine' and 'archaic' are some of the descriptions heard in medical circles. However, I hope to explore some of the evidence pointing to the spiritual dimension of people and its place in a holistic perspective of health.

REFERENCES

1 WHO. www.who.int/about/en/
2 *The Concise Oxford Dictionary of Current English*. 9th ed. Thompson D, editor. New York: Clarendon Press; 1995.
3 Smuts JC. *Holism and Evolution*. Gouldsboro: Gestalt Journal Press; 1996.
4 Dummer T. *Tibetan Medicine and Other Holistic Health Care System*. New Delhi: Paljor; 2002.
5 Oltmans TF, Emery RE. *Abnormal Psychology*. New Jersey: Prentice Hall; 2000.
6 *BMJ*. 2004; **329**(7473): front cover.
7 CRAP Writing Group. EBM: unmasking the ugly truth. *BMJ*. 2002; **325**: 1496–8.
8 Spence D. Evidence-based medicine can lie. *Doctor*, 24 June 2004.
9 Hippocrates. *On airs, waters, and places*. Translated by Francis Adams, 1849.
10 Dickens C. *Bleak House*. First published 1852–53.
11 Howden-Chapman P, Matheson A, Crane J, *et al*. Effect of insulating existing houses on health inequality: cluster randomised study in the community. *BMJ*. 2007; **334**: 460–4.

12 BMJ poll. Medical Milestones. *BMJ*. 2007; **334**: s2.

13 Longmore M, Wilkinson I, Rajagopalan S. *Oxford Handbook Clinical Medicine*. Oxford: Oxford University Press; 2004.

14 Locker D. *Symptoms and Illness: the cognitive organization of disorder*. London: Tavistock; 1981.

15 Morris D. *Illness and Culture in the Postmodern Age*. London: University of California Press; 2000.

16 Austen J. *Mansfield Park*. 1814.

17 Austen J. *Persuasion*. 1817.

18 Gelder M, Harrison P, Cowen P. *Oxford Textbook of Psychiatry*. Oxford: Oxford University Press; 2000

19 Coni N, Davison W, Webster S. *Lecture Notes on Geriatrics*. 3rd ed. London: Blackwell Scientific Publications; 1988.

20 Brontë C. *Shirley*. Ware: Wordsworth Editions; 1993.

21 Austen J. *Sense and Sensibility*. 1811.

22 Ader R. *Psychoneuroimmunology*. 4th ed. New York: Academic Press; 2008.

23 Ader R, Cohen N. Behaviorally conditioned immunosuppression and murine systemic lupus erythematosus. *Science*. 1983; **214**: 1534–6.

24 Cohen S, Frank E, Doyle WJ, *et al*. Types of stressors that increase susceptibility to the common cold in healthy adults. *Health Psychol*. 1998; **17**(3): 214–23.

25 Cohen S, Doyle WJ, Turner RB, *et al*. Emotional style and susceptibility to the common cold. *Psychosom Med*. 2003; **65**: 652–7.

26 Persky VW, Kempthorne-Rawson J, Shekelle RB. Personality and risk of cancer: 20-year follow-up of the Western Electric study. *Psychosom Med*. 1987; **49**(5): 435–49.

27 Pietroni PC. The meaning of illness – holism dissected. *J R Soc Med*. 1987; **80**(6): 357–60.

28 Balint M. *The Doctor, his Patient and the Illness*. London: Tavistock; 1957.

29 Sontag S. *Illness as Metaphor*. New York: Viking; 1979.

30 Rousseau J-J. *Confessions*. London: Penguin Books; 1973.

31 Graves R. *The Greek Myths*. London: Penguin Books; 1992.

32 Holmes OW. The new century and the new building of the medical school of Harvard University. *Boston Med Surg J*. 1883; **109**: 361–8.

33 British Holistic Medical Association. www.bhma.org/modules.php?op=modload&name=PagEd&file=index&topic_id=0&page_id=50

34 General Medical Council. *Good Medical Practice*. London: GMC; 2006.

35 Mattson P. *Holistic Health in Perspective*. Mountain View: Mayfield Publishing; 1981.

36 Scott I. *What Will It Take? A Deeper Approach to Nature Conservation*. West Hoathly: HPT Books; 1999.

37 Sachs J. Survival in the Anthropocene. Second 2007 Reith Lecture given at Peking University, Beijing, China, April 2007. www.bbc.co.uk/radio4/reith2007/lecture2.shtml#lecture2

38 Ho M-W. *Genetic Engineering – Dream or Nightmare: turning the tide on the brave new world of bad science and big business*. 2nd ed. London: Continuum International Publishing Group; 2000.

39 Campo R. *The Other Man Was Me: a voyage to the New World*. Houston: Arte Publico Press; 1994.

40 White P. What can general practice learn from complementary medicine? *Br J Gen Pract*. 2000; **50**(459): 821–3.

41 Diamond J. *Snake Oil and Other Preoccupations*. London: Vintage; 2001.

42 Baum M. Paying a complement: should the NHS fund alternative medicine? *The New Generalist*. 2006; 4(3): 26–7.

43 Lewith G. Should complementary medicine be made available on the NHS? www.complemed.co.uk/articles/index.htm (accessed on 09/02/09).

44 Linde K, Clausius N, Ramirez G, *et al*. Are the clinical effects of homeopathy placebo effects? A meta-analysis of placebo-controlled trials. *Lancet*. 1997; **350**: 834–43.

45 Shang A, Huwiler-Müntener K, Nartey L, *et al*. Are the clinical effects of homoeopathy placebo effects? Comparative sudy of placebo-controlled trials of homeopathy and allopathy. *Lancet*. 2005; **366**: 726–32.

46 Eastwood H. Complementary therapies: the appeal to general practitioners. *Med J Aust*. 2000; **173**: 95–8.

47 Radley DC, Finkelstein SN, Stafford RS. Off-label prescribing among office-based physicians. *Arch Intern Med*. 2006; **166**(9): 1021–6.

48 NICE. Insomnia – newer hypnotic drugs. http://guidance.nice.org.uk/TA77

49 Freeman J. Towards a definition of holism. *Br J Gen Pract*. 2005; **55**(511): 154–5.

50 EURACT. European definition of General Practice/Family Medicine, www.woncaeurope. org/Web%20documents/European%20Definition%20of%20family%20medicine/ Definition%20EURACTshort%20version.pdf

51 Charlton BG. Holistic medicine or humane doctor? *Br J Gen Pract*. 1993; **43**(376): 475–7.

52 Hasegawa H, Reilly D, Mercer SW, *et al*. Holism in primary care: the views of Scotland's general practitioners. *Prim Health Care Res Dev*. 2005; **6**: 320–8.

53 Wilson T, Holt T, Greenhalgh T. Complexity science. *BMJ*. 2001; **323**: 685–8.

54 Encyclopaedia Britannica. www.britannica.com/eb/article-9105912/complexity

55 Leader D, Corfield D. *Why do People get Ill?* London: Hamish Hamilton; 2007.

56 Schlaegel TF. *Psychosomatic Ophthalmology*. Baltimore: Williams & Wilkins; 1957.

57 Astin J, Astin W. An integral approach to medicine. *Alt Ther Health Med*. 2002; **8**(2): 70–5.

58 Shakespeare W. *The Tragedy of King Lear*. 1603–6.

59 Lamb C, Lamb M. *Tales from Shakespeare*. 1807.

CHAPTER 2

Are we spiritual?

'Music is the movement of sound to reach the soul...'
Plato

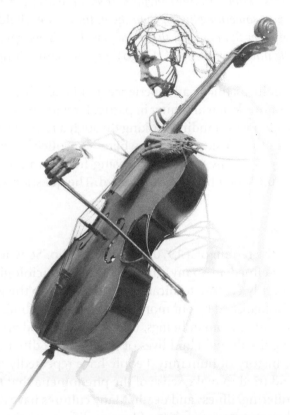

Cellist by Lau Hung

'We are not human beings on a spiritual journey. We are spiritual beings on
a human journey.'[1]

Pierre Teilhard De Chardin

Debates about the existence of God have raged for thousands of years. Theists on one side argue that the source of the universe is the Creator while atheists hold the view that there is no God and that religion is pure mythology or the 'opium of the people' as Karl Marx said so famously. Distinguished philosophers and scientists have seen evidence for theism in the structure of the physical world while equally eminent scholars – and Richard Dawkins comes to mind – view religion as a refuge of the unthinking and the malevolent, and that those who argue for it are either knaves or fools.[2] I suspect that debates like this will continue for as long as time lasts with neither party thoroughly managing to convince the other – at least with its argument. Anyway, I regard this as all rather academic because I am more concerned about the everyday experience of everyday people. I doubt that anyone is capable of proving irrefutably that we do *not* have a spiritual dimension, especially as this would be at odds with what many experience in their own lives.

The statements: *'I am certainly convinced that it is one of the greatest impulses of mankind to arrive at something higher than the natural state'* (Baldwin)[3] and *'There is one spectacle grander than the sea, that is the sky, there is one spectacle grander than the sky, that is the interior of the soul'* (Hugo)[4] say the same thing. They attest our spiritual nature.

I remember quite distinctly an experience that I had which on retrospect was spiritual. I do not think that anything in particular had provoked it. I must have been about six and I was standing looking through a rain-spattered window on to the greyness of the outside. From nowhere – unsolicited and surreptitiously – a question crept into my mind, as if arising from an inner part of me with which I had up until then been unacquainted. The question was, 'Who am I?'

WHO ARE YOU?

'Who are you?' is the refrain of a 1970s hit by The Who. So who are we? Human beings may be defined in many different ways – sociologically, anthropologically, biologically etc. Anatomically we are related to the great apes but we are reputedly distinguished by our more highly developed brain with its capacity for abstract reasoning. Human beings, the world and God are three important areas permeating the thought and lives of people from different cultures, races and eras in the history of humanity. People have repeatedly asked themselves who they are and tried to make sense of the phenomena that they observed, of their lives, of suffering, illness and death. Many cultures have always recognised an incorporeal or spiritual principle of human life or existence corresponding to the soul. Many believed that this soul has an afterlife. It is enough to stroll through the British Museum to have an idea of how central the spiritual is throughout time – from the dazzling contents of the tombs of Ancient Egyptians to an exhibition of pieces from China's Terracotta Army, which the First Emperor constructed to guard him in the next life.

Ancient Greeks – particularly Plato – had a dualist view of reality and the identity of the human being did not derive from the body but from the character of the soul. For Platonists the soul was a spiritual substance akin to the gods and yet part of the changing world. Epicureans instead believed that the soul consisted of atoms like the rest of the body. René Descartes considered human beings a union of the body and the soul – each a distinct substance having some action on the other while Benedict de Spinoza thought that the body and soul formed two dimensions of a sole reality. At the beginning of the twentieth century, William James held that the soul did not exist but was a collection of psychic phenomena. The American defence lawyer Clarence Darrow also denied its existence:

'If there is a soul, what is it, and where did it come from, and where does it go? Can anyone who is guided by his reason possibly imagine a soul independent of a body, or the place of its residence, or the character of it, or anything concerning it? If man is justified in any belief or disbelief on any subject, he is warranted in disbelief of a soul. Not one scrap of evidence exists to prove any such impossible thing.'

Clarence Darrow (1857–1938)

There may be no hard evidence for the existence of the soul but there is no shortage of dictionary definitions: the spiritual or immaterial part of a human being often regarded as immortal.[5] Whether or not we choose to believe in the existence of the soul, Jung considered that we are bound to it.

'People will do anything, no matter how absurd, in order to avoid facing their own souls.'

Carl Jung (1875–1961)

A SOUL QUEST

In the late 1960s a scientist set out to explore if a spiritual dimension (and therefore the soul) does exist. He obtained results that surprised him. This scientist was Sir Alister Hardy. Formerly professor of Zoology at Oxford University, Hardy founded the Religious Experience Research Unit in 1969 – now called the Religious Experience Research Centre (RERC). Hardy, a Darwinian and self-defined inquiring naturalist, was not of any religious persuasion but he was convinced that our spiritual dimension was in some way linked with the evolutionary process. The Research Unit was concerned with understanding spiritual feelings and the effect these have on our lives. *The Spiritual Nature of Man*, published in 1979, was based on the first eight years' work of the unit. It drew on thousands of first-hand accounts the unit collected from individuals. Some of these accounts describe the spiritual dimension:

I think that from childhood I have always had the feeling that the true reality is not to be found in the world as the average person sees it. There seems to be a constant force at work from the inside trying to push its way to the surface of consciousness. The mind is continually trying to create a symbol sufficiently comprehensive to contain it, but this always ends in failure...[6]

For some time I have experienced myself an extraordinary contact with what I may call some 'power' or guidance outside my ordinary day-to-day life...but in some unexplainable way my long search for 'light' seems to be leading me towards what I most need. I can now contact the vast storehouse of power that comprises the universe. By concentrated, voiceless prayer and, in a way, relaxation, I may feel my whole spirit filled with this power, and my whole being recharged. When this happens, then I know that anxiety, troubles and so forth will be solved; and indeed they are.[6]

Hardy[6] observed that the dogma of materialism makes a growing number of people regard the idea of a spiritual or transcendental aspect of the universe as a pleasing illusion or myth remaining from a pre-scientific age which civilisation must supersede. Hardy questioned materialism as the sole lens through which we are able to view the world and why consciousness, 'the seat of all our values' is ignored in the equation of life. He attempted to classify the spiritual experiences that he collected from the research participants. Some experiences were sensory, some behavioural and some cognitive.

Some of the cognitive elements were:
➤ a sense of security, protection and peace
➤ a sense of joy, happiness and well-being
➤ hope and optimism
➤ a sense of new strength in oneself
➤ a sense of release from fear of death
➤ a sense of guidance, vocation and inspiration
➤ a sense of purpose behind events
➤ a sense of presence (not human).

Study participants spoke of triggers to spiritual experience such as music, art, natural beauty, literature, depression, solitude, childbirth, illness, bereavement and the prospect of death. The internationally renowned neuropsychiatrist Peter Fenwick has studied near death experiences and dying over a number of years. He has collected many accounts of the dying who have experienced a deep sensation of love and light during the passage from life to death. There are other reports of people feeling the powerful presence of a loved one who, unbeknown to them, at that moment was dying elsewhere. There are no rational, scientific explanations for these phenomena. They do not tally with a mechanical, material world-view. They would however suggest that the consciousness is not entirely based in the brain and that it can exist when the brain stops functioning. Something – soul or consciousness – continues beyond death.[7]

Torrance[8] observes that setting out on a spiritual 'quest' is characteristic of our humanity and that as a species we could with equal justification be called homo 'quaerans' as well as homo 'rationale'. He defines this quest as the deliberate effort to transcend the given limits of the human condition and notes that it is a universal phenomenon typical of the tribal peoples of West Africa, Central Asia or the Amazon. We find it in the shamanistic processions of Japan, in the

> restless search for the Taoist islands of immortality, 'in the pilgrimages to Benares, Jerusalem, Mecca or Rome; or in the mystical aspirations of Muslim Sufi….But there could be no greater provinciality, no narrower ethnocentrism, than to think the questing spirit a monopoly of the Faustian West or an innovation of the Great World Religions. It is far more deeply rooted and more widely spread.

THE SPIRITUAL DIMENSION AND EDUCATION

Society is managed by systems – social, economic, political, legal – and the spiritual dimension could seem extraneous to the smooth running of daily life. However, our education system recognises the importance of the spiritual dimension in its young charges. One of the areas that OFSTED (Office for Standards in Education) evaluates is the spiritual, moral, social and cultural development of pupils – in other words, it takes an all-rounded approach to education. Although acknowledging that it is difficult to define spiritual development, particularly in a setting where there are people of religious or non-religious affiliation, it does nevertheless try to do so. The 1994 inspection handbook states:

> Spiritual development relates to that aspect of inner life through which pupils acquire insights into their personal experience which are of enduring worth. It is characterised by reflection, the attribution of meaning to experience, valuing a non-material dimension to life and intimations of an enduring reality.[9]

An OFSTED discussion paper[10] defined the following as features of spiritual development:
- beliefs
- a sense of awe, wonder and mystery being inspired for example by the natural world, mystery or human achievement
- experiencing feelings of transcendence.

OFSTED recognises that the search for meaning and purpose and the 'why me?' at times of hardship and suffering are other facets of the spiritual dimension, as are reflecting on the origins and purpose of life and its challenging experiences such as beauty, suffering and death. The National Curriculum Council considers spiritual development so important that without it children 'would live in an inner spiritual and cultural desert'.[11] OFSTED provides a description of spiritual development that attempts to be very inclusive. It says the spiritual dimension is the

> non-material element of a human being which animates and sustains us and, depending on our point of view, either ends or continues in some form when we die. The spiritual dimension is concerned with a sense of identity, self-worth, personal insight, meaning and purpose. It is about a person's spirit. Some people would call this the 'personality' or 'character'. Others would call it a person's 'soul'.[12]

Spiritual development is about how pupils address 'questions which are at the heart and root of existence' and it is identified as 'the idea of the spiritual quest, of asking who you are and where you are going'.[12]

Again, the idea of the quest echoes Torrance's earlier description of the human race as homo quaerans.

Quests have always fascinated us – from Homer's *Iliad* to Tolkien's *Lord of the Rings*. In *The Pilgrim's Progress*[13] the main character, Christian, is in a deep spiritual crisis. To save his soul he embarks on a spiritual journey to the Celestial City. He overcomes many difficulties on his journey – such as the Slough of Despond and imprisonment in the Doubting Castle – to reach eventually the City. Christian journeys through the wilderness, which is symbolic of an inner struggle and the arduous path the soul must follow every day. Through such quests, we face the great existential questions, which have haunted and harried people from the beginning of time: what does my life mean? who am I? where am I going? We are not any different from our predecessors who inhabited the earth. There may be greater technology and questionably more 'sophistication' and 'civilisation' but our fears are still the same. There are many questions about ourselves that we cannot answer. There is much about us that is mystery. Myths, legends, and quests somehow resonate with something within us. It is enough to look at the box office success of films such as the Matrix trilogy and the Star Wars series.

LESSONS FROM THE ARTS

Literature and art reveal the existence of our spiritual nature. In fact, DH Lawrence in 'Making pictures'[14] says that it needs a certain 'purity of spirit' to be an artist and the motto, which should be written over every School of Art, is: 'Blessed are the pure in spirit, for theirs is the kingdom of heaven'. He explains that being pure in spirit is the 'beginning of all art, visual or literary or musical'. It is not the same as goodness for him but 'more difficult and nearer the divine'.

There is something in us that makes us feel that we are more than we appear to be and that our spirit goes on forever. Such were possibly the sentiments of Steven Cummins, a soldier killed in Northern Ireland. He left a poem in an envelope to be opened in the event of his death. This poem was the most sought after in the BBC's favourite poems of the nation competition. The poem speaks about the writer's spirit continuing after death in the wind, glinting sunlight and 'the swift uplifting rush of quiet birds in a circled flight'.[15]

Emily Dickinson's poem has different interpretations, one being the triumph of the spirit over death:

> Death is a Dialogue between
> The Spirit and the Dust.
> 'Dissolve' says Death – The Spirit 'Sir
> I have another Trust' –
> Death doubts it – Argues from the Ground –
> The Spirit turns away
> Just laying off for evidence
> An Overcoat of Clay.
>
> Part Four: Time and Eternity, XXXI[16]

The artist's 'purity of spirit' is evident in many works. From time immemorial, we have gazed with awe at the wonders of our surroundings and inferred that some divine power was behind it all:

> Tyger! Tyger! burning bright
> In the forests of the night
> What immortal hand or eye
> Could frame thy fearful symmetry?
>
> In what distant fires or skies
> Burnt the fire of thine eyes?
> On what wings dare he aspire?
> What the hand dare seize the fire?[17]

When writers wish to express some of the 'deepest and most elusive elements' about our spiritual nature, they often use animal imagery.[18] Such is the case in *Watership Down*[19] and the Duncton Chronicles.[20] *Watership Down* is about the search by a group of rabbits, led by Hazel, for a new home. The rabbits overcome adversity, betrayal and hardship to reach eventually their 'promised land'. The

Duncton Chronicles trilogy is a fantasy about religious conflict and a kingdom of moles whose life centres on the standing stones and stone circles of Britain.

They say the eyes are the mirror or window of the soul. By looking into someone's eyes, you sometimes have an idea of the type of person who is in front of you. Eyes speak. They mirror sadness, joy, pain, disappointment, fear and some inner presence. One of my friends works for an NGO and she went recently to visit a tribe in a remote part of Kenya. The people were adamant about not having their photographs taken – they felt that their souls were being 'captured' on camera and they did not relish the thought!

Perhaps cameras do trap the spiritual. The BBC launched a project called 'Divine Art' where participants could send in pictures, which inspired them spiritually. A contributor sent in a photograph of a sky window of a deer shelter.[21] Some of the visitors to the deer shelter had a spiritual experience when they looked up at the sky window. One of the comments was 'superbly contemplative' and 'more spiritually fulfilling than most art' and another person focussed on how looking at the window had given a sense of being uplifted to a higher plane.

Lau Kwok-Hung is a present-day Chinese artist. His sculptures simulate Chinese calligraphic brushstrokes but closer examination reveals an intertwining network of iron rods that form dynamic human figures. Hung overlays his sculptures drop by drop with molten iron and his work varies from dancing figures to figures playing a symphony together. He does not complete his figures, yet each one is 'an emblem of earthliness as well as transcendence'. The magical, 'empty' space is an invitation to the viewer to 'penetrate the interplay between concept and realization in pursuit of clues to the very meaning of existence'.[22] However, for Hung – like many artists – when a work is complete, it is already obsolete, because the artist cannot live 'without continuously creating...without this insatiable urge to express what his soul demands be made manifest'.[23]

Some of our best literary works focus on our spiritual nature. Oscar Wilde's Dorian Gray is beautiful and this results in a Faustian pact: he offers his soul in return for perpetual youth. While his beauty remains unblemished, his portrait ages and becomes loathsome. In some way it mirrors the depravity of his soul. In the culminating moment of the story, Dorian says the soul 'can be poisoned or made perfect. There is a soul in each one of us. I know it.'[24]

CS Lewis' books have fascinated and continue to fascinate an endless number of children and adults. Perhaps one reason for their attraction is the spiritual themes, which permeate them. In his personal life, he fought hard against belief in any higher being. During his first years at Oxford University, logic obsessed him. It seemed to be the only consistent force in a meaningless universe. His argument against the existence of God was the cruelty and unjust nature of the world but then he began to question the basis for this argument. He considered that if life is truly meaningless how could he possibly know this, given that he would have no sense of what meaning actually is? It would be analogous to a fish complaining it was wet when it has no concept of dry or a man calling a line crooked when he has no concept of a straight one.[25] He mused that creatures are not born with desires unless satisfaction for those wishes exists. A baby feels hunger and in response food satisfies, a duckling wants to swim and water is available to serve the purpose: 'If I find in myself desire which no experience in this world can satisfy, the most probable explanation is that I was made for another world.'[25] He called this desire

> the secret signature of each soul, the incommunicable and unappeasable want, the thing we desired before we met our wives or made our friends or chose our work, and which we shall still desire on our deathbeds. While we are, this is. If we lose this, we lose all.[26]

Lewis described another spiritual experience:

> We do not want merely to *see* beauty. We want something else, which can hardly be put into words. We want to be united with the beauty we see, to pass into it, to receive it into ourselves, to bathe in it, to become part of it. At present we are on the wrong side of the door. We discern the freshness and purity of morning, but they do not make us fresh and pure. We cannot mingle with the splendours we see. But it will not always be so. Some day, God willing, we shall get in.'[27]

For Lewis there is no such thing as 'ordinary people'. Nations, cultures, arts, civilisations are mortal but 'it is immortals who we joke with, work with, marry, snub and exploit – immortal horrors or everlasting splendours'.[27]

Music can be a strong communicator of the spiritual – from the music of Bach to soul music that originated from black Gospel music. The French composer Olivier Messiaen wrote 'Quartet for the End of Time' (*Quatour pour le fins du temps*). The German army captured and detained him as a prisoner of war during World War II. Within the setting of this dismal blank hell, uncertain whether he would ever see his family or all that he loved again, Messiaen wrote this quartet, which speaks of transcendence, light and eternal joy. His fellow captives – a cellist, violinist and clarinettist – used their dilapidated instruments to play the piece, transfixing guards and prisoners alike in a profound spiritual experience.[28] Messiaen, who also had the rare gift of synaesthesia, able to 'see' sound as colours, was an 'intensely spiritual' man. For him, even birdsong was a code for transcendence.[29]

SPIRITUALITY AND THE MODERN AGE

What is spirituality? The word is actually French Catholic in origin but the reality existed thousands of years before this. In fact, up to now I have chosen to avoid the word 'spirituality' in order to focus on the spiritual dimension itself. There is also much confusion about the word 'spirituality' and the difference between spirituality and religion. When 'ity' is added to a word to form a noun, it denotes 'quality or condition' or 'an instance or degree of this'. I prefer to think of spirituality as an 'instance' or an illustration of the spiritual dimension.

For some the term spirituality is analogous to religion and for others it embraces everyone with or without a religious affiliation. Spirituality is described as a vast realm of human potential dealing with ultimate purposes, with higher entities, with God, with life, with comparison and with purpose.[30] Shafranske and Gorsuch describe spirituality as 'the courage to look within and trust. What is seen and what is trusted appears to be a deep sense of belonging, of wholeness, of connectedness and of openness to the infinite.'[31] Another definition of spirituality is 'that which is involved in contacting the divine within the self – 'self' referring to the realms of consciousness well beyond the ego and individual perceptions of faith'.[32]

Benor concludes the great diversity found in the usage of the word suggests to some 'the concept is hopelessly vague and thoroughly unsalvageable for scientific use'.[33]

Some argue that 'spirituality' as used in the modern New Age context is something subjective, without any reference to a higher authority and with reliance on the inner authority – hence the move away from established religion.[34] Major bookstore chains have sections labelled 'Mind Body and Spirit' or similar words and such literature has jumped from 0.9% of the total market in 1998 to 5.8% in 2003. Alternative therapies are all often thought to be 'spiritual'. For Heelas and Woodward, astrology, chiropractics, flower essences therapy, herbalism, palm reading and nutritional therapy are examples of 'holistic milieu activities'.[34] There is an illustration from a local newspaper in Heelas' book,[34] promoting the idea that 'holistic therapy' is spirituality: a client lies prone on a couch and a complementary therapist is giving him soothing aromatherapy massage. The caption reads 'alternative spirituality is growing fast…' Words such as 'balancing', 'well-being', 'therapy' seem automatically to be endowed with holistic properties regardless of the product on sale and – seeming 'holistic' – they are deemed spiritual.

During the late 1960s in British life, in tandem with what was happening in the States, there was a renewed interest in spiritual issues. LSD and other drugs were used to explore consciousness and there was a quest for transcendence. The discovery then followed that the 'spiritual' effects induced by drugs could be induced by other methods such as meditation, yoga, sensory deprivation, fasting and dancing. Leech outlines that there was a reversion to primitive forms of 'spiritual journey' such as witchcraft, astrology and occult movements. He thinks the pop music of the time and even the musical 'Hair' were vibrant with this search for meaning. The new-found interest in the eastern religions – particularly in Buddhism and Zen Buddhism – also flourished.[35]

There were three characteristics of this spiritual journey during the sixties and to some extent, these themes endure today: disenchantment with the conventional established religions of the West, especially with institutionalised Christianity, desire for transcendence and deeper ways of experiencing reality and concern for peace, justice, human liberation and fulfilment.[35] The awakened interest in spirituality occurred against the background of great changes: political, social and cultural. Charlene Spretnak attempts to unravel the mystery behind what she calls the recovery of meaning in the postmodern age. She highlights the failure of the cult of modernity to deliver its promises of peace, freedom and fulfilment on condition that we would discard our 'embarrassingly superstitious' past.[36]

Spretnak depicts ours as 'an age of fading utopian dreams and looming utopian nightmares'.[36] She also speaks of crises: the external crises of modernity (destruction of the natural world, the nuclear race, exploitation of the developing world and indigenous peoples for the demands of industrialised nations and 'homo oeconomicus') and the internal crises, which includes a search for meaning in our lives and respite from a sense of isolation. Other aspects of these crises are the impoverishing of human culture, the incapacity to reason morally and the deterioration of community and family ties.

The failure of modernity has led to the search of new or the recovery of old meaning: new meaning in the understanding of nature and the connection between our species and the rest of the natural world. Spretnak elaborates on the two remedies that have evolved to fill the vacuum created by this lack of meaning. There is the phenomenon of 'deconstructive post modernism', expressions of which may be intense cynicism, denial, indifference and disengagement, and 'ecological post-modernism' which is constructive or reconstructive. Ecological post modernism recognises that all beings are intrinsically inter-connected – even at the molecular level.

Araujo, a sociologist, describes how the quest for meaning is occurring at a hectic pace and that even the media takes advantage of this:

> In front of the TV, in the comfort of your living room, the sacred…is offered as a mixed dish at a buffet: a little pinch of Islam, a slice of esotericism, a drop of transcendental meditation with, according to your personal taste, a little bit of Christianity, sprinkling of sects, Buddhism…and, voilà, fast food nectar that produces 'emotions' and 'sensations', poor substitutes for what every person in every age searches for: happiness. In this search of the happiness for which they yearn, people of today trust themselves to the care of magicians, witches, palmists, astrologers. They search for the unknown in and beyond the stars.[37]

If spirituality is authentic, it surely must be more than just a manufactured, consumable commodity. It must be something that helps us live the experience of life, death and suffering: something that truly gives meaning. In his post-mortem of modern society, Leech suggests that we are located in a terrible space and in a new Dark Age. For him 'the only spirituality which can suffice is one which will provide us with the resources to survive and to outlive the prevailing darkness.'[38]

Renetzky gives a definition of the spiritual dimension, which I favour because I find it workable:

> The 'power within man' giving 'meaning, purpose and fulfilment' to life, suffering and death; the individual's 'will to live'; the individual's belief and faith in self, others and God.[39]

Spirituality concerns the sense of meaning and purpose of life – it concerns issues such as illness, death, suffering – life in its light and shadows. People have been 'about spirituality' for thousands of years. Spirituality has found expression in myriad ways according to different religions, cultures, history, social structures and life events. Spiritualities are as diverse as the contemplative prayer of the sages of Asia to the joyful African spiritualities. Who would dispute the spiritual grandeur of people such as Mahatma Gandhi, Martin Luther King or of the figure on the front cover of a 2007 edition of *Time* – Mother Teresa of Calcutta – described as 'as one of the great human icons of the past 100 years'?

In this chapter, I have tried to demonstrate that we are not simply biological beings but homo 'quaerans' on a spiritual quest. This spiritual dimension is recognised in the Arts and Education, even though the rational world of science often does not consider it relevant or even existent. We seek for the meaning of our lives – inevitably touched by illness, suffering and death – often through our spiritual dimension.

The next chapter explores the link between the spiritual dimension and health.

REFERENCES

1 www.dictionary-quotes.com/we-are-not-human-beings-on-a-spiritual-journey-we-are-spiritual-beings-on-a-human-journey-pierre-teilhard-de-chardin/
2 Haldane J. 'In the crossfire'. *The Tablet*. 24 November 2007.
3 Baldwin J. The male prison, nobody hears my name. In: Tripp RT, editor. *International Thesaurus of Quotations*. Middlesex: Allen & Unwin; 1987.
4 Hugo V. *Les Miserables* (*Fantine*). Wilbour C, translator. In: Tripp RT, editor. *International Thesaurus of Quotations*. Middlesex: Allen & Unwin; 1987.
5 *The Concise Dictionary*. 9th ed. Thompson D, editor. Oxford: Clarendon Press; 1995.
6 Hardy A. *The Spiritual Nature of Man: a study of contemporary religious experience*. Oxford: Clarendon Press; 1979.
7 Fenwick P, Fenwick E. *The Art of Dying*. London: Continuum; 2008.

8 Torrance RM. *The Spiritual Quest: transcendence in myth, religion and science*. Berkeley: University of California Press; 1994.

9 Handbook for the Inspection of Schools. Part 4. Inspection Schedule Guidance. Consolidated edition. HMSO; 1994.

10 Ofsted. Spiritual, moral, social and cultural development: an Ofsted discussion paper. Ofsted; 1994: 8.

11 Spiritual and moral development – a discussion paper. York: National Curriculum Council; 1993.

12 Ofsted. Promoting and evaluating pupils' spiritual, moral, social and cultural development. 2004. Accessed at: www.ofsted.gov.uk/Ofsted-home/Publications-and-research/Browse-all-by/Education/Curriculum/Religious-education

13 Bunyan J. *The Pilgrim's Progress*. Oxford: Oxford University Press; 2003.

14 Lawrence DH. Making pictures. In: Boulton JT, editor. *DH Lawrence: Late Essays and Articles*. Cambridge: Cambridge University Press; 2004.

15 Anonymous. Do not stand at my grave and weep. In: *The Nation's Favourite Poems*. London: BBC Worldwide; 2006.

16 Dickinson E. *Complete Poems*. 1924.

17 Blake W. *The Tyger*. 1794

18 Wakefield G, editor. *Dictionary of Christian Spirituality*. London: SCM Press; 1996.

19 Adams R. *Watership Down*. London: Puffin Books; 1973.

20 Horwood W. *Duncton Wood. Duncton Quest. Duncton Found*. London: Arrow Books; 1985, 1989, 1990.

21 www.bbc.co.uk/bradford/content/articles/2007/01/04/divine_brian_deer_shelter_feature.shtml

22 Hung LK. Ten Thousand. Brochure produced by Atelier Hung. Valdarno; 2006.

23 www.atelierhung.com/English/dossier/dossier.GB.html

24 Wilde O. *The Picture of Dorian Gray*. London: Penguin Books; 1994.

25 Lewis CS. *Mere Christianity*. London: HarperCollins; 2002.

26 Lewis CS. *The Problem of Pain*. London: HarperOne; 2001.

27 Lewis CS. *The Weight of Glory*. London: HarperCollins; 2001.

28 Rischin R. *For the End of Time: the story of the Messiaen Quartet*. Ithaca: Cornell University Press; 2006,

29 Morton B. 'Traveller beyond time'. *The Tablet*. 16 February 2008.

30 Tart C. *Transpersonal Psychologies*. Law Book Co of Australasia; 1975.

31 Shafranske E, Gorsuch R. Factors associated with the perception of spirituality in psychotherapy. *Journal of Transpersonal Psychology*. 1984; **16**: 231–41.

32 Fahlberg L, Fahlberg L. Exploring spirituality and consciousness with an expanded science: beyond the ego with empiricism, phenomenology and contemplation. *Am J Health Promot*. 1991; **5**(4): 273–81.

33 Benor DJ. *Healing Research: holistic energy medicine and spirituality: volume one*. Munich: Helix Editions; 1993.

34 Heelas P, Woodhead L, Seel B, *et al*. *The Spiritual Revolution: why religion is giving way to spirituality*. Oxford: Blackwell Publishing; 2005.

35 Leech K. *Soul Friend: a study of spirituality*. London: Sheldon Press; 1977.

36 Spretnak C. *States of Grace: the recovery of meaning in the postmodern age*. London: HarperOne; 1991.

37 Araujo V, Dreston A, Rossé G, *et al*. Dio Amore nella tradizione cristiana e nella domanda dell'uomo contemporaneo. Rome: Città Nuova Editrice; 1992 (author's translation).

38 Leech K. The Shape of Babylon: the political context of spirituality. In: Robson J, Lonsdale D, editors. *Can Spirituality Be Taught?* London: Association of Centres of Adult Theological Education and British Council of Churches; 1985.

39 Renetzky L. The fourth dimension: applications to the social services. In: Moberg D, editor. *Spiritual Well-being: Sociological Perspectives*. Washington: University Press of America; 1979.

CHAPTER 3

The neglected dimension of health

'He that has light within his own clear breast/May sit in the centre, and enjoy bright day: But he that hides a dark soul and foul thoughts/Benighted walks under the mid-day sun; Himself his own dungeon.'

John Milton

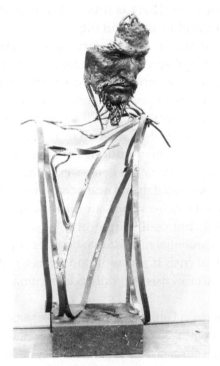

Blind Saul by Lau Hung

THE NEGLECTED DIMENSION

In ancient times in many traditions, medicine was considered a gift of the Divine. In Egypt, Bast the cat deity was thought to confer health and happiness. Thoth, with the head of an Ibis and the body of a man was the god of learning, wisdom, healing and medicine. The ancient Greeks believed that Athena had revealed medicine to humankind. Medicine was a calling to a deep transformation in the sick person and to true conversion. The healing of the body was an effect of the healing of the soul obtained through purification and catharsis: the re-establishment of a spiritual relationship with the divine re-established balance – that is, health. In the Mesopotamian and Egyptian cultures, being sick was associated with sin and so illness was perceived as punishment. Egyptian papyri describe the course of various illnesses but they also describe monthly purification ceremonies. Religious ritual seems to have been essential.[1] Over centuries, the spiritual dimension in medicine diminished in importance.

Although there is an increasing awareness now of the value of the spiritual aspect, this recognition has been slow to appear in today's medicine. However, there are signs. About ten years ago, an article in the Lancet affirmed that the spiritual dimension was gaining support in the USA.[2] At present there is an ongoing debate about the effects of religious and spiritual factors on health, illness, prognosis and healing. There is much empirical data on the beneficial effect of religion on morbidity and mortality.[3,4,5]

The words of Trevor Smith, a psychiatrist and homeopathic practitioner, strike me profoundly. He observes that because of our capacity to think, our existential awareness and concern centres on faith, morals, philosophy, our belief in ourselves and the meaning and purpose of our existence. We are fully aware of our transience, vulnerability and fragility and because we feel as if we are a tiny particle in a vast hole 'rather than of being that whole', we may ultimately feel alone – sometimes without the language to articulate what we actually experience or question. Smith defines existential malaise as the 'feelings of despair and loneliness, inevitability and acceptance, albeit wary acceptance, that accompanies such awareness and...an intrinsic part of the uncertainty of the questions, seemingly impossible to resolve'.[6]

Speaking about the existential malaise that besets many people, he expresses his concern that this spiritual crisis is just as important as any industrial, inflationary, unemployment or monetary crisis, but only gets minimal media coverage:

> In almost every home in Europe or the U.S. families sit night after night, unselectively watching 'rubbish' on the television. Usually they are watching contrived programmes, which are of no interest to them: they are glued to the set, not thinking, not talking, passive...and it is not the fault of the television, it is a symptom of our society...[6]

Philosophy is one of the subjects not generally taught to children in British schools – unlike the experience of their peers in other European schools. A lack of familiarity with philosophising may make it difficult to articulate and cope with some of our innermost feelings. Eventually we *do* have to do some philosophising in our lives, especially when earth-shattering events overtake us and we are faced with questioning the meaning of our existence.

Socrates said the unexamined life is not worth living. Unfortunately, many of us live this type of life today. We get up, have our breakfast, dress, eat, go to work, have our lunch break, continue to work and then go home. We eat again, exchange a few words with family or friends, watch TV, change for bed, fall asleep and repeat the same routine seven, ten, or more, thousand days in our lives rarely stopping to reflect on who we are, what is important to us, where we are going and who we wish to become. The unexamined life is one that is lived at some level almost like a somnambulist on automatic pilot – a life based on values and beliefs that we have never really looked at, tested or examined for ourselves. Philosophy helps us examine life and is 'map-making for the soul'.[7]

Smith[6] argues that the great impulse is to drive out thought and to become oblivious to any deeper questioning. Existential malaise leads to an increase in existential anxiety for many people resulting consequently in a rise in mental and physical illness. For Smith, the ability to accept a degree of 'not knowing' and uncertainty about life is the 'culmination of health' and having the resilience to bear doubts and anguish is a test of maturity. Smith wrote his book twenty years ago and of course since then there has been much talk of 'spirituality' to the extent that a few years ago, *Cosmopolitan* appointed a spirituality editor. *The Times* reported that this appointment was made in response to the needs of the readers who felt a hole in the soul and were not satisfied with their lives despite having everything they materially wanted.[8]

However wanting a quick fix to fill this hole is not the answer either if it fails to help us face the widespread moral and spiritual crisis highlighted by contemporary European philosophers, such as Camus, Kierkegaard and Sartre, and poetry such as the Rubáiyát. The urgent rush and need to be impulsively involved in any new fad, therapy, religion, diet or gadget the media can most plausibly put over as a 'good' can be itself a symptom. It may be a symptom of the failure to engage deeply with the existential crisis that we all must face as we mature as human beings. Integrating this spiritual aspect of our nature is an important part of our health. Smith further comments that the presence of mental and physical illness may reflect underlying denial and suffocation of the unavoidable existential challenge.[6]

Aristotle claims that the purpose (*telos*) of human beings is to attain happiness – an activity of the soul linked to virtue. Happiness for him is not just sensual pleasure (he considered this a view fit for grazing cattle) but rather genuine happiness is a by-product of living in a way conducive to the deepest human flourishing for ourselves and for others.

Morris believes there are four universal dimensions of human experience that help us understand the four corresponding targets we need to aim at if we are to attain and promote happiness in our own lives and in the lives of others. These four dimensions are the intellectual, the aesthetic, the moral and the spiritual.[7] Morris considers that while the first three dimensions are concerned with truth, beauty and goodness respectively, the spiritual dimension encompasses 'unity, inner unity, unity between myself and others, between all human beings and the rest of nature and, ultimately, between nature and nature's source'. For people of religious affiliation, nature's source is God.

Everyone has spiritual needs. They need:
➤ uniqueness
➤ union
➤ usefulness
➤ understanding.[7]

Spiritual needs are too deep for us to put temporarily aside for the sake of some other good. We may choose to neglect or ignore them and if we do so, it is to our detriment.[7]

Uniqueness is the need to feel special and distinct. At its most trivial, it might be expressed by wearing or doing something 'different' just to stand out in a crowd. At its most exalted, it is the feeling that in the history of humanity there only ever will be one me.

Union is the sense of being united to something greater than the self such as the family, community, the world, humankind, God.

Usefulness is the need for creativity, the sense that we are on this earth for a purpose. Hence, unemployment is not just an economic problem but also a spiritual one. I spent some time in a developing country where many of the young people are unemployed. They are desperate for education; they go to university so that they can get jobs, then they graduate and find there is virtually nothing for them. They will do the most menial of tasks – anything – to work. One of these young people wrote to me to tell me how happy he was at working in a warehouse. He was not able to use his biology degree but at least he had a steady job and he was grateful for that. Work is not simply about earning – work is about our creativity and dignity. Whether we are house-parents, high-flying chief executives or lying ill in bed we still need to feel useful, creative and that we have a purpose.

The fourth spiritual need is the necessity to feel a 'deep emotional **understanding** of our place in the world'.[7]

Meeting spiritual needs improves our well-being and therefore our mental health. Health Scotland is a national agency for improving the health of the people of Scotland. On its website, there is a definition of mental health that recognises the importance of the spiritual dimension:

> Mental health is a generic term, which describes an integrative approach embracing affective, behavioural, cognitive, physiological, socio-political and spiritual health.[9]

A definition of spiritual well-being is a state of acceptance of self and others with a positive disposition towards life and a sense of harmoniousness and connectedness between self, others, nature and the ultimate 'other'. This inter-connectedness exists beyond time and space and is achieved through a dynamic integrative growth process leading to the realisation of the ultimate purpose and meaning of life.[10]

Koenig and his co-authors[11] looked extensively at research on religion and health. They found that people not affiliated to any religion were at greater risk of depressive illness and symptoms while those who valued their religious faith were at a reduced risk of depression and tended to recover more quickly. They also discovered that religious involvement was linked to a greater sense of well-being and life satisfaction, a greater ability to adapt to bereavement, lower rates of suicide, less anxiety, less psychosis and lower rates of alcohol and drug abuse. Studies have demonstrated that depressive symptoms and an absence of personal meaning are more common in those with a weak to a moderate faith in a transcendent power, while those with a strong belief are better 'protected'.[12]

In the section labelled 'other conditions that may be a focus of clinical attention', DSM-IV, the Diagnostic and Statistical Manual of Mental Disorders, recognises a new category – neither psychological nor pathological – entitled 'Religious or Spiritual Problem'.[13] It gives as examples distressing experiences that involve loss or questioning of faith and questioning of spiritual values not necessarily related to an organised church or religious institution – evidence again of the importance of the spiritual dimension.

The spiritual dimension of a person is like a beverage that has different characteristics. It might resemble the bubbly effervescence of a carbonated drink or the mellow velvet of a long matured glass of wine. The literature and research on the spiritual dimension and medicine has been increasing in latter years especially in the field of palliative care. However, the spiritual dimension may be evident in many aspects and stages of the lives of patients, carers and health professionals alike.

SPIRITUAL HEALTH AND OLDER PEOPLE

In the Eastern and African cultures, old age has tremendous spiritual value and elders are crowned with a halo of sacredness. Buddhists too welcome a long life. For Hindus the disabilities and frailties of the mind and body have a purpose: they are an aid to development, the opportunity to move on to another sphere. Old age is all about wisdom and according to the writer Robertson Davies, 'a truly great book should be read in youth, again in maturity and once more in old age, as a fine building should be seen by morning light, at noon and by moonlight'.[14]

Cicero has some glorious words to say about old age and, although two thousand years separate us, his words to his friend Scipio poignantly reveal their spiritual dimension. He regards earth as a 'place of entertainment' and not of residence and looks forward to the day when he will leave this world and join 'that heavenly conclave and company of souls'. He recalls the death of his son Cato whose funeral pyre he had torched and the consolation that the parting and separation between them would not be for long. For this reason, his old age 'sits lightly on me and is not only not oppressive but delightful'. However, he also says, 'If I am wrong in thinking the human soul immortal, I am glad to be wrong; nor will I allow the mistake which gives me so much pleasure to be wrested from me as long as I live.'[15]

William Wordsworth rather romantically extols old age describing a woman in her seventieth year as if the years had put her through some sort of distilling process and produced a refined distillate of 'something purer and more exquisite'. He compares her to a 'welcome Snowdrop' with 'temples fringed with locks of gleaming white, and head that droops because the soul is meek'.[16]

In the West there is sometimes a fear of old age, often regarded as devoid of any purpose. There is a fear too of the illnesses that may accompany it. Jack Coulehan is stark in his description of Irene – a stroke victim – and her difficulty with communication:

After the third stroke,
her words fell off
to a few soft syllables…

With what looks like weakness,
she wobbles
her left hand to my wrist,
but that grip
is the grip of a woman
who clings by a root
to the face of a cliff.
When she speaks, her words
are small stones
and loosened particles
of meaning
that tumble to their deaths
before my ear
is quick or close enough
to save them. *Irene,*
tell me again, I say,
after the words
in her bits of chopped breath
are gone. But George
takes his cap from my desk
and puts it on his head, and says
Her gulps don't make no sense.[17]

Old age with the loss of health, independence and bereavement that it brings, can result in spiritual crisis. It does not take much to imagine that Irene, stricken with stroke, faces such a crisis and George too, in his own way. He reduces his wife's words to 'gulps' thus making her sound like a desperate animal, something subhuman.

The following example is typical: a woman loses her 63-year-old husband prematurely from cancer and then enters deep depression. For the first time she starts to ponder about things previously taken for granted. She questions her religious beliefs and her doubts disturb her. A lecture hosted by Age Concern looked at how this 'secular organisation' should respond to spiritual need in the twenty-first century. It was recommended the organisation have knowledge of the diversity of spiritual beliefs of older people. Other recommendations given were respect for spiritual beliefs and discernment of the spiritual needs of older people.

Spiritual need may be intense and hidden when a sudden illness takes away activity, interests and the very meaning of existence. Eveline is typical of the many older people we see in hospital wards, residential care and in their own homes:

> I am 85 years old and became a widow many years ago. I have had a very active life, had my hobbies, went to concerts and the theatre. My days were always full. All of this until I reached my eightieth year. That evening I felt well. There were all the normal ailments of age, but nothing that foretold what was to happen the following day. In fact, the day after I ended up in hospital with heart problems, problems with the brain, the stomach and the dorsal spine. It was as if my whole body had collapsed from one moment to the next. They patched me up pretty well, but that day my life was turned upside-down. I was now a chronic invalid. It tired me to speak, to read, to walk. I could only vegetate and gulp down medicine. I experienced boredom, depression and frustration at having to suddenly abandon all my activity! I continued to repeat to myself: but what am I still living for, what use am I to anyone now?
>
> One thing that greatly bothered me was the attitude of my children. Before we had a beautiful relationship of great trust, now they didn't tell me anything that was happening. Poor dears! They were certainly trying to be considerate, but it all gave me a sense of solitude, of marginalization.
>
> I suffered badly – perhaps more spiritually than physically.

Eveline found peace and came to terms with her illness when she was able to face her spiritual pain and give it meaning. She was able to embrace old age and its attendant problems gracefully. In approximately 500 BC, Pindar said that a graceful old age is the childhood of immortality[18] and childhood too has a spiritual dimension.

SPIRITUAL HEALTH AND CHILDHOOD

A couple brought their newborn baby boy home and presented him to his four-year-old sister. One night the little girl asked if she could talk to her baby brother all by herself. Though thinking that this was rather odd, her parents agreed. They left the little girl alone with her brother and listened in another room with the baby monitor. As they listened from the other room, through the monitor they heard the child whisper to her brother, 'Tell me about God before I forget.' This story seems bizarre, but not to some scientists. Justin Barrett is a researcher at Oxford University on the cognitive science of religion. His research suggests that children have a natural default belief in God – belief at odds with the view that belief is learned from indoctrination within the family. Children appear to be 'wired for God'.[19]

Death, any suffering, impacts on the life of a child and therefore on a child's health.[20] People who work with children need to recognise that sometimes it may be important and appropriate to focus on religion and the spiritual dimension. A healthcare worker recounts a sad story – the premature death of a young mother and its effect on her daughter. The mother had tried to bring up her children amid terrible adversity but she had also made mistakes in her life. The girl worries about her mother's soul: would she be judged as harshly in the afterlife as she was here on earth?[21]

For more than thirty years, Robert Coles has extensively researched the spiritual life of children. He was professor of psychiatry and medical humanities at Harvard University. He originally had a scientific view of his young clients that regarded as irrelevant any reference made to anything spiritual, let alone religious. The children themselves challenged this position in unspoken words that went much like this:

> Doctor, I was told, you're not interested in my religion, only my problems. But without my religion, I'd be much worse off, don't you see? How about encouraging me to talk about that movie, about what I experience when I go to church, instead of sitting bored, waiting for God to pass from this conversation?...about trying to learn what I've learned as a child at home, church, at Sunday school, so that you will be able to respond to me rather than to some paradigm, of which my mind and its workings seem to be for you a mere illustrative instance?[22]

Coles worked with many children who did not consider themselves religious and did not attend any form of organised worship. They shunned such descriptions as 'utterly inapplicable to themselves'. These children asked many spiritual questions about the nature and meaning of this life:

> You take the kids whose folks aren't into any religion; we have lots of them in our school, and they're no different than anyone, and some of them – I talk with them

about what they believe – are really great, because they ask a lot of questions about life, and they want to stop and talk about things, about what is right
and wrong, and what you should believe, and after I'll talk with them, I'll say to
myself, hey, maybe if you have no religion, you end up being more religious. You
know what I mean?[22]

If literature is 'the lie that tells the truth'[23] by simplifying and heightening reality then the creation of alternative worlds may help us confront some of life's
deeper questions. *The Lord of the Rings*, the Narnia and Harry Potter books are
such examples. According to Francis Bridger,[24] the spirituality and morality of
the three famous friends of Hogwarts – Harry, Ron and Hermione – promote the
all-conquering power of love. Harry survives a destructive curse of the evil Lord
Voldemort because of the traces of the self-sacrificial love of his mother, which
still protect him.

Bridger goes on to illustrate that many of the characters display the same
self-sacrificial love: Lupin and Sirius Black, Harry, Hermione, Ron and yet again
Harry. At one point Harry physically stands in the way of the death of the man
responsible for his parents' murder – at risk even to his own life. In fact, Row-
ling 'would seem to embrace self-sacrificial love as something of a credo – a
moral philosophy to live by'.[24] Potterworld is not just a series of adventure books
with tremendous appeal to children and adults alike but it has become a true
cultural icon, successfully translated into many diverse national and sub-
national cultures…it connects with something intrinsic to the human spirit.[24]

Anna is another child depicted in literature. However, unlike Harry Potter
who is fictitious, *Mister God*'s Anna *did* exist. Fynn[25] found the waif-like Anna
wandering the grim streets of East London at a time when foundlings were not
uncommon. Anna was like a rainbow that Fynn captured in his hands but she
was no ordinary child. At five years old, she had a degree of depth and wisdom
that many people do not carry even into their old age. She knew the purpose of
being and the meaning of love. Her spiritual dimension was precocious – she
died before her eighth birthday – and yet it was not abstract but something real
and tangible: 'after a few weeks of Anna the street and the people in it took on
a buttercup glow'.[25]

'Mister God' was very real to Anna. After an explanation from Fynn about a
yellow flower absorbing all the colours of the spectrum apart from yellow, which
is reflected back to the viewer, Anna concluded that yellow was reflected back
because the flower did not *want* this colour. Anna gives her own explanation
about why people cannot see 'Mister God'. A flower that does not want the
yellow light is called yellow and that is what we see. Whereas, 'you couldn't say
the same thing about Mister God. Mister God wanted everything, so he didn't
reflect anything back. Now if Mister God didn't reflect anything back, we
couldn't possibly see him, could we?' For Anna, Mister God was quite empty. He

did not have the emptiness of non-existence but the emptiness that accepted everything, made everything and everyone welcome and did not reflect anything back!

Perhaps one of the hardest things in life is to see a child suffer. Images of children in war-torn or famine-stricken countries move many of us. It might be the photograph in a leaflet of a child with tears coursing down her dirty cheeks, eyes questioning why she is suffering and seeming to look directly at you. There are other images. It might be the toddler who kicks furiously while he is held down for an injection. It might even be the unutterable, unuttered suffering of a child not safe in his own home. Suffering might bring with it some sort of spiritual crisis. It might even be the first time that the child meets this aspect of his or her life. Suffering might serve as a catalyst for spiritual crisis and growth. Suffering, angry children – just like adults – might find themselves saying:

> 'When there's a storm, I always stop and listen. If there was a God, He'd be say-ing something! I don't think there is one, though. I've tried to pray; I've asked why my little brother was born with that disease; why he suffers so much, why he won't live a normal life; why he'll probably die when he's young, the doctors say. That's not fair; that's not justice – for a boy to be sick, always, with colds, and his lungs don't work right. When we took Joey to the hospital the other day, he seemed brave. He said whatever happens will be all right with him. I wasn't happy at all! I saw a priest come and pray for the kids, and I wanted him to come over to our room and explain why it's so unfair, what happens, and why, if people pray to God, He doesn't answer their prayers a lot of the time. My brother has seen such misery in his life – hospital so many times, and each time he comes back with terrible stories: you just can't imagine how bad it can be for some people! Does God know about all this? – I'd like to know!'[22]

Zattoni and Gillini write that the sufferings of a child – the child we all bear within ourselves – will not be devastating if they are given a meaning and if we do not fall into the trap of trying to explain everything away.[26] They direct this message to all people who in some way have contact with children – the parent, carer, teacher, doctor, nurse... The authors have experienced that children have strategies for healing themselves. The first strategy is to distance themselves from the source of the pain, the second is to enjoy the agreeable things that life con-tinues to offer and the third is to look suffering in the face. They warn against the temptation to overprotect children or to over identify with their suffering to the extent that they feel that they are unable to cope:

> Our culture...seems always to be teaching...that suffering should be banished as if it were a great obstacle. We have been conditioned to think that where there is

suffering something must be wrong and therefore the old idea of training ourselves to face suffering is somehow out of date... The idea that growing up, matur-
ing or simply living in this world necessarily involves suffering is something we are
conditioned to resist with all our might. And yet, if we do not learn to accept times
of suffering as part and parcel of growing up, we shall find ourselves – albeit involuntarily – saying no to life itself.[26]

Some adults do not feel comfortable around children and I have often wondered why. Perhaps one of the reasons is that because of their honesty and sim-
plicity, they have the untrained knack of getting to the truth and telling you the
heart of the matter, just like the Little Prince. He bewails the fact that grown-ups
think they learn something about others from figures (their weight, earnings,
age etc). Yet the secret that the fox told the Prince encapsulates the spiritual life
of children: 'You can only see clearly with your heart. Your eye cannot see what
is essential.'[27]

THE SPIRITUAL DIMENSION AND MENTAL HEALTH

Psychiatrists are increasingly recognising the importance of acknowledging and
encompassing the spiritual dimension of their patients. Since 1999, the Royal
College of Psychiatrists has had a Special Interest Group, which looks at spirituality and psychiatry. The group offers a forum for psychiatrists to explore the
spiritual dimension of patients and psychiatrists alike. At the time of writing, the
membership of the group numbers over 1600. The inspiration behind forming
the group was the patron of the College, HRH Prince Charles. Already several
years before, he had encouraged the College to adopt an approach embracing
the mind, body and spirit.

In a survey of 210 US family doctors about attitudes toward spiritual health,
68% believed that strong religious convictions positively influence the mental
health of older people while 42% believed such convictions have a positive
effect on physical health.[28]

The Mental Health Foundation undertook a survey in 1998 and this showed
that over 50% of service users hold religious or spiritual beliefs that they see as
valuable in helping them cope with mental illness. The survey also highlighted
the need that many patients feel for encouragement in discussing these concerns with their psychiatrists. The Special Interest Group has held seminars with
titles as varied as 'Spiritual Issues in Child Psychiatry' to 'Invited or not, God is
here: spiritual aspects of the therapeutic encounter'.[29]

The Royal College of Psychiatrists also produces a leaflet for patients on
spirituality and mental health. Patients consider the benefits of paying attention to their spiritual health to be:

➤ improved self-control, self-esteem and confidence

➤ faster and easier recovery, achieved through the promotion of healthy grieving over loss and the maximising of personal potential
➤ improved relationships with self, others and God/creation/nature
➤ a new sense of meaning, resulting in the reawakening of hope and peace of mind, enabling people to accept and live with problems not yet resolved.[29]

The Spirituality Special Interest group also considers 'reciprocity' to be an important principle of the spiritual approach to mental healthcare where the giver and receiver both benefit from the interaction. These are some of the skills that it considers spiritual:
➤ being self-reflective and honest
➤ being able to remain focussed in the present, remaining alert, unhurried and attentive
➤ developing greater empathy for others
➤ finding courage to witness and endure distress while sustaining an attitude of hope.

The spiritual health of the patient is not just the realm of the palliative care team or of the psychiatrist. Psychologists and psychiatrists have spoken of the disturbances in mental health, which they have noted in people when the spiritual dimension is not nurtured. Ionata writes of how Frankl describes as noogenic the neurosis, which arises from a lack of value and meaning in life. Maslow prefers instead to talk of 'metapathology' where people are deficient in transcendent values. In 1932, Carl Jung made the clinical observation that the prevalence of neurosis was linked to the decline in religious practice. He felt there was a serious lack of balance in the general spiritual state of Europeans and that this was responsible for a confused, unsettled and agitated way of looking at life. He found that a large percentage of his clientele consulted him not because of true neurotic illness, but because they were unable to find any meaning in their lives. They were tortured by problems, where they had found no answer in philosophy or religion.[30]

In his book *Man's Search for Meaning*, Frankl describes his horrific experiences in a concentration camp and his psychotherapeutic method of finding meaning in all forms of existence – even the most unbearable situations. Born into a Jewish family in Vienna, after medical school he specialised in neurology and psychiatry. In 1942, he was deported to Auschwitz with his wife and parents. In concentration camps, he worked in both the psychiatric and neurological units, trying to care for his fellow inmates who were weary of life. His own experiences and the sufferings of others in such harrowing conditions made him conclude that even in the most adverse circumstances, life has potential meaning and therefore suffering is meaningful too.

After the Second World War, Viktor Frankl founded Logotherapy, considered the third Viennese school of psychotherapy. In logotherapy, the psychologist takes into account the client's search for meaning and therefore the spiritual dimension. The psychotherapeutic approach is based on three philosophical and psychological concepts:

➤ freedom of will
➤ will to meaning
➤ meaning in life.

The assumptions of logotherapy, like all psychotherapies, can neither be proved nor disproved with certainty, but to see if they make sense in our lives we have to assume that they are true. According to Frankl, freedom is the space to shape one's own life within the limits of given possibilities. This freedom stems from the spiritual dimension of the person. When a person cannot fulfil his or her 'will to meaning', there is an empty meaninglessness. The frustration that results leads to aggression, addiction, depression, suicide and it may result in or aggravate psychosomatic complaints and neurotic disorders. Logotherapy does not offer some general meaning in life, but it does assist clients in achieving 'the openness and flexibility that will enable them to shape their day-to-day lives in a meaningful manner'.[31]

Elisabeth Lukas is one of Frankl's most noted students and founder of the Institute of Logotherapy. She became interested in logotherapy because she was disillusioned with learning about human behaviour by studying the behaviour of rats – 'rat psychology' – with the philosophy that people were animals and could be treated like research specimens. Frankl appealed to her because he addressed the spiritual dimension. She concedes that although we can neither prove nor disprove the existence of the spiritual dimension, its importance lies in the approach it allows us to adopt with patients. We can see them either as incorrectly programmed computers or as people who can transform suffering into something greater.

Lukas explains the approach she would give to a patient who feels that a huge mountain is blocking his path. This mountain might be depression, anxiety, dependence on something or someone or an inferiority complex. For her, the traditional psychologist concentrates on the obstacle and asks why it is there, who put it there, how it can be gradually decreased – but this does not help overcome the obstacle. Instead, logotherapy asks what is so important and precious that it can make a person go beyond the obstacle. Logotherapy helps the patient look not so much at what has gone badly within him or herself but rather at the most beautiful thing that he or she contains. Only after this does the therapist begin to look with the patient at the problems.

Logotherapy could therefore be confused with spiritual care but Lukas argues that although they are quite distinct, they could be mutually beneficial. Those who provide spiritual care often are unaware that problems are not actually religious but psychosomatic and vice versa.

Logotherapy has implications for health promotion, as people who have found a meaning to their life are psychologically sound. Lukas has also used it with relaxation techniques, meditation, conventional medicine, grief counselling and when patients have to face loss such as the diagnosis of a terminal illness. In Canada, the logotherapeutic approach was used in a large project to help preserve the indigenous Indian culture, while medical students in South American universities learn to quote pages of Frankl's work. Logotherapy however is not a panacea. It is difficult to apply logotherapy when patients are under the influence of drugs or are in serious psychotic states and cannot express the spiritual dimension so easily.[32]

THE SPIRITUAL DIMENSION AND HOMEOPATHIC MEDICINE

As previously suggested, there is the idea that everything 'alternative' in alternative medicine is spiritual. However the absence of matter in a given therapy does not necessarily mean that it involves anything spiritual. It would be like saying that radiotherapy is spirituality simply because you cannot see it or equally that oxygen therapy is spiritual. Yet some of the alternative therapies can encompass the spiritual dimension. Examples are spiritual healing and some aspects of homeopathic medicine.

I first started to practise homeopathic medicine with what I think was healthy scepticism. I still maintain some degree of scepticism towards this and conventional medicine. In fact, perhaps it is a good idea to be healthily sceptical in medicine generally because ultimately we can never be one hundred per cent certain that what *we* are doing is the principal factor that makes a particular person better. Homeopathic medicine seemed very woolly to me and in some respects uncomfortably unorthodox. How could it possibly work with its ultra-molecular doses and with medicines that seem to be prescribed sometimes at the whim of the prescriber rather than using a reproducible scientific approach?

'Homeopathy-bashing' is nothing new. Almost a hundred and seventy years ago, Sir Oliver Wendell Holmes, gave a lecture on 'Homeopathy and its Kindred Delusions'. He pointed out, 'Homeopathy has proved lucrative, and so long as it continues to be so will surely exist – as surely as astrology, palmistry, and other methods of getting a living out of the weakness and credulity of mankind and womankind.' He further said

> ...so long as the body is affected through the mind, no audacious device, even of the most manifestly dishonest character, can fail of producing occasional good to those who yield it an implicit or even a partial faith'.

However, what Holmes found even more ridiculous is the vague belief that 'matter subdivided grows less material, and approaches nearer to a spiritual nature.[33]

Should you ask a homeopathic practitioner to justify his therapy he will commonly say that Hippocrates considered there were two principles of treatment in medicine: the Law of Opposites and the Law of Similars. The first principle is the one that forms the basis of conventional Western medicine. If someone has a temperature, you give a drug that lowers the temperature; if someone suffers from insomnia, you give a drug to induce sleep. Hahnemann and the first homeopaths used the Law of Similars to treat illness. They gave Belladonna – the deadly nightshade – to help the patient with a high temperature, flushed face and hallucinations. Belladonna poisoning causes a dry mouth, thirst, fever, dilated pupils, hallucinations... However, Belladonna could not be given unmodified because of its toxicity. Therefore, the homeopaths diluted the substances that they used – often toxic – and then shook them vigorously at each stage of dilution. They found that these dilutions still worked. Oddly, they should have been inert if we reason according to the knowledge of science that we have today. These medicines should not have worked because, unknown to the homeopaths, the substances sometimes were being diluted beyond 'Avogadro's number' (that is beyond a stage where there was a miniscule – if any – material presence of the substance). 'Nothing' was there!

Didier Grandgeorge, a French homeopath, explains the process like this: 'The 'material' substance disappears leaving in place the message, the spirit of that substance.' (Wendell Holmes's precise criticism!) He argues that this is undoubtedly due to what certain audacious and courageous scientists such as Poitevin and Benveniste have called 'water's capacity for memory'. Water, and above all water mixed with alcohol seems able to 'seek out, copy, and transmit the information contained in the dissolved substance much as the iron filing retains the imprint of a magnetic field even when the magnet is taken away'.[34] Could this paradox be true and dismantle some of what we understand of science? Does it not simply reflect what physicists observe today and cannot fully understand: behaviour at the particle level is frustratingly unpredictable? Who would have believed a hundred years ago the devastation unleashed by splitting a humble atom? Homeopaths consider that their clinical experience verifies that something *is* at work – something more than 'placebo'.

The debate on homeopathy – and on many complementary therapies – still rages. In the West, homeopathy will never gain serious credibility among doctors today unless there are many more positive trials – of the randomised controlled variety.[35] However, if homeopathy is simply a placebo effect then it is evidently a very superior placebo since animals and babies – to whom homeopathy is often administered effectively – respond.

As I treated more people with homeopathy, I had to set aside some of my scepticism and concede that I obtained results that I could not explain – results that I could not dismissively attribute to the 'placebo effect'. The best results were those achieved in the most cynical patients or in young children where there was little chance of a placebo effect. For example, there was the hyperactive toddler who would not sleep. He tore around his room tirelessly for much of the night. His mother came desperately to see me. I tried a homeopathic preparation of Chamomilla, which resulted in his sleeping after an hour. This was already a considerable improvement but I felt that we could do better. I then tried homeopathic Coffea and after taking this, he slept within a few minutes. His mother was delighted! Then there was the boy with the facial tic. This problem had occurred in the past and had resolved only after several months. I tried homeopathic Agaricus and within a week, the tic had gone. Of course, the results could have been the effect of mere coincidence. The bizarre thing is I have consistently seen many 'coincidental' positive results with homeopathy. If you are curious to test out homeopathy, it is worth applying Arnica cream to a bruise or take 6C or 30C tablets twice daily for a few days. Afterwards observe if the bruise resolves any quicker than usual.

I have to admit, however, that what first aroused my interest in homeopathic medicine were not the theories about how it works or some aspects of the 'science' of homeopathic medicine with which I still struggle but the approach of the homeopathic practitioner to the patient. I often found in the courses that I attended such enthusiasm among the doctors – enthusiasm that I had not even noticed at medical school. In homeopathic medicine the approach is truly holistic. Every aspect of the patient is important, or potentially important: how he looks at you, his shyness, his pathology, how it affects him, his fear of death, his fear of the supernatural, his spiritual immaturity, his preoccupation with too much of the 'spiritual' – everything. In fact, many practitioners would probably agree with the words of a homeopath:

> When we don't deal with issues on the spiritual, mental and emotional, they will then break through into the physical plane.[36]

Hahnemann, the founder of modern-day homeopathy, spoke about the 'vital force' that he regarded as some form of spiritual energy in the person.[37] Kent, a great teacher of classical homeopathy, essentially perceived the root of many illnesses was spiritual.[38] Vithoulkas, a renowned present-day homeopath, divides the human being into three arbitrary levels: the physical, emotional and mental/spiritual level. For him, the mental and the spiritual content of the person is the true essence of the person.[34] He summarises the definition of the health of the whole person as:

➤ freedom from pain in the physical body – having attained a state of well-being
➤ freedom from passion on the emotional level – having as a result a dynamic state of serenity and calm
➤ freedom from selfishness in the mental sphere – having as a result total unification with Truth.

Vithoulkas does not define what he means by 'Truth' but he sees it as something transcendent. Nevertheless, he does specify that the parameter, which enables such a holistic measurement of health, is creativity:

> By creativity, I mean all those acts and functions which promote for the individual himself and for others their main goal in life: continuous and unconditional happiness.[39]

The description which Gray, a leading American homeopathic practitioner, gives of a skin condition that he successfully treated is typical of the potential for deep healing that exists in homeopathy.[40] Gray looked at the patient on all three levels – physical, emotional, mind/spiritual – considering her feelings of low self-esteem following the breakdown in her marriage. After treatment with the indicated homeopathic medicine, not only did the skin condition heal but the patient also reported a great change in her life. She became more assertive, confident and happier.

The only explanation of this cure with the biomedical model is again a placebo response, and yet homeopathy has been shown to be superior to placebo.[41] A meta-analysis performed at the University of Limberg did show that of the 107 controlled homeopathy trials that were reviewed, 81 demonstrated positive effects while 24 lacked positive results.[42] Although the authors considered the favourable outcomes may have been due to publication bias in the trials that they studied, they agreed there was a legitimate case for further evaluation of homeopathy using 'well performed trials'.

Classical homeopathic medicine aspires to look for the unique medicine for each unique patient. Unlike the doctor who has a choice of analgesics or anti-inflammatory medication for arthritis and varies the prescription according to patient tolerance of side effects, the possible interaction with other drugs and of course the efficacy of the drug, in homeopathic medicine it is quite different. In classical homeopathy, the practitioner will look for the homeopathic treatment which best matches not just the patient's symptoms and their characteristics but also he might consider food preferences and – even odder – his personality.

Many homeopathic medicines could potentially help haemorrhage, however the homeopath looks at the 'whole' picture of the patient for guidance in the remedy choice. The following is a case from several decades ago which benefited from Ustilago maidis. The homeopath took into account the haemorrhage and hair loss:

> About a fortnight before Hurndall saw the patient she had aborted five foetuses, at about the fifth week of gestation. Since then there had been passive haemorrhage of dark clots. Moreover, she was a perfect specimen of alopecia, not having a hair of any sort on her body and only a little about the head. Us. 3x

(Ustilago maidis, 3x potency) was prescribed, five drops three times a day. In two days the haemorrhage was completely arrested, tenderness reduced, spirits revived, and general health improved. At the end of three months, there was a nice coat of hair growing, which in due course became perfectly normal.[43]

This case was not that of a woman but of a small dog.

Ustilago is a fungus known as corn smut and was adopted as a homeopathic medicine after the discovery that animals feeding on the smut tended to abort, shed their hair or lost their teeth. In homeopathy, it may be used for menorrhagia, fibroids, problems with the nails, alopecia, a history of miscarriages and during the menopause.

George Vithoulkas[44] describes how a patient's emphasis of the spiritual dimension may be valuable in identifying the homeopathic medicine appropriate for him as with Aurum metallicum (gold) prepared homeopathically. Clinical experience has shown its usefulness in complaints as varied as testicular problems to depression. Vithoulkas comments that some patients who benefit from Aurum are 'very proper and moralistic' and they may display excessive 'religious behaviour', with a tendency to 'pray constantly for salvation'.

People who need a homeopathic medicine from the Cactaceae family may present at the latter stages of their lives where at best all a practitioner can do is accompany them in their search for a meaning to their existence. 'Cactaceae patients' for example may be extremely hypochondriacal, destroying their own life and the lives of the people around them because of their incessant demands and complaints. They sometimes do not trust in any relationship – even with their doctors – and they do not even totally trust their medicines. Fascinatingly when they become seriously ill, they seem 'relieved' as if their long-standing fears of having a serious illness have finally been justified. It is as if they have now found their true identity as a sick person, with all its 'rights and privileges'. Ironically, instead of being frightened, they are more serene. Their illness provides another way of escaping and of avoiding contact with the world around them.[45] However, at the end of their lives, such people may reach a spiritual understanding of life. They are even able to trust deeply and seriously in God, but in their own specific way. They do not necessarily feel an affiliation to any particular religion, but they may have a private spiritual approach to life and to their illness. Their words and behaviour may betray this since they do not willingly divulge it.[40]

I remember a patient who was tremendously anxious about his health. He would come for the least thing – always convinced there was something seriously wrong with him. Nothing would ever pacify him and he seemed to leave the surgery barely reassured...until he came back with the next symptom. This had gone on for years with other doctors. Finally, I received a hospital letter following a discovery of a serious condition, which proved to be terminal. I was afraid for the patient because, given his over-anxious personality, I imagined that he would not be able to cope. He amazed me when I next saw him. I had never seen him so serene and with such inner peace. At the time, I was not familiar with homeopathic medicine, otherwise I could have helped him even further – possibly with a homeopathic medicine from the Cactaceae family. Instead of just stopping at his anxiety, through taking a homeopathic history I would have tried to discover what lay behind it.

Calcarea carbonica may help problems with respiratory tract infections, constipation, eczema and nightmares. It is a homeopathic medicine often given to children. According to Vithoulkas, between the ages of six and twelve they commonly develop an intense curiosity about spiritual things, the unknown and what lies beyond. They may ask questions such as 'What is God? Why do people die? What happens to us after death?' Of course, many children ask these questions and I remember asking myself those questions at that age. However, Vithoulkas considers that in these children the curiosity and fixation about the spiritual is so powerful that you may find them actually waiting for an angel to come to take them to paradise.[44]

I AM ALWAYS THINKING THAT I AM DYING OF SOMETHING…

Nitricum acidum is another homeopathic medicine, which may benefit patients who are very anxious about their health. These people may greatly fear death and the thought of not existing. Every little illness or even the 'symptoms' provoked by their normal physiology are harbingers of death. Their fears are existential.

Amanda is a 35-year-old woman who I treated with homeopathy. Incorporating her spiritual dimension and her existential fears led to my prescribing the homeopathic remedy to which she responded very well. She suffered from IBS – irritable bowel syndrome. During the session, I did not offer any counselling. I simply let her tell her story:

> I get quite bad indigestion when I pass wind very frequently and it is quite painful at times. I go to the toilet regularly and I am quite often constipated. The cyst (ovarian) is quite big. I am always thinking that I am dying of something and it overtakes my life… I am always the one who is going to be ill and leave my daughter. I am afraid of getting cancer and I don't go out in to the sun. Almost every morning I check my skin. I have had counselling and I try… At the moment we are all healthy and every day I try to be positive but I have heard so many terrible stories – a business friend of my father died at 49 of a heart tumour, a little girl at school died of leukaemia at nine. Everywhere I look…when I hear about illness or death I have to leave the room.
>
> I know I am going to die one day but not now…the whole cancer thing…the chemo, losing your hair, the stories that I have read about people writing diaries

when they have had cancer and been treated for it. I feel I am often unhappy or stressed and something.

I was convinced I was HIV positive at 18 … There was all this advertising that I saw. Things just blow out of all proportion.

I had a pain inside and said to the doctor I had cervical cancer. It is not bad every single day but in general there is this cloud where you just think.... It is difficult to feel happy sometimes. It is illness and recovering from illness – but more important it is leaving my daughter behind with no mother.

I am not sure if I worried as a child. I did I think. I was bullied at school and used to be sick on a Sunday but they found out it was because of this.

I wake up at night worrying about things – work or money and not so much illness. I probably dream but I don't really remember them. When I first had my daughter, I dreamt that I died and I went in to this black hole thing. This big bus ran over me and I went into oblivion...this black hole.

I get butterflies in my tummy until I have been to the doctor. If I do have anything, I cannot really relax until I have been to the doctor. I don't feel happy. If I am happy about something, I can be brought down to earth by the thoughts [of death]. If I die, I want it to be sudden. I don't want to have to suffer torment and get treatment and know I might die. I feel unhappy now when there is nothing really wrong with me…

…I had postnatal depression. I found it difficult – she whinged a lot. I wondered if I had done this [had a child] too early. If I got pregnant, again I would be so worried about the risks involved…

…My husband thinks I worry too much. He does say I am a worrier. I often think I am a terrible mum because I am racing around. I worry about other people and how she behaves. If she is naughty when we are out and does not say 'please' and 'thank you' then I can get disappointed in her.

Amanda's anxiety about her health is obvious from her story. This anxiety has a large impact on her life: 'I am always thinking of dying of something and it overtakes my life…I am afraid of getting cancer and I don't go out in to the sun. Almost every morning I check my skin.' She had daily thoughts about death triggered often by the slightest thing. She knew that she was being irrational but she could not stop the thoughts overwhelming her. Amanda had tried counselling but to no avail. As I was taking her history, I realised that her fears were really existential. She could articulate how she felt incredibly well but she could not fathom what her fears actually meant. I suspect that she never really asked herself the question and perhaps she did not wish to know the answer.

Words such as '…I dreamt that I died and I went into this black hole thing. This big bus ran over me and I went into oblivion…' and, 'If I die I want it to be sudden. I don't want to have to suffer torment and get treatment and know I might die,' betrayed her fear of not existing, of the unknown, of suffering. This existential fear and the fear of suffering (in other words her spiritual dimension) which underpinned her anxiety made me prescribe Nitricum acidum. She responded very well to this medicine.

Follow-up at two months: Amanda reported that she was less anxious about her health. She was able to reassure herself now that she did not have anything wrong with her: 'Even the thought of illness is not coming into my head.' She started to notice the improvement shortly after beginning Nitricum acidum. The IBS also improved.

Review at seven months: She was still doing well and no longer had any real anxiety about death. She was able to push her anxieties to the back of her mind and volunteered that they were no longer uncontrollable. Amanda's job was stressful but she felt able to cope.

Review at 11 months: Amanda commented: 'Taking the homeopathic medicine has completely changed my life...I no longer have all-consuming thoughts about death.'

When Amanda came for review sixteen months and then two years following her first appointment, she was still much better despite 'having the occasional blip'. At no point had she been on any conventional medication, nor was she having any form of counselling. The IBS was still better. She self-rated her improvement at +3 (large improvement that has a major effect on daily living) in the Glasgow Homeopathic Hospital Outcome Score (GHHOS). GHHOS is an instrument to measure patient's views of the outcome of their care by asking them to describe the impact on daily life.[46]

Aristotle says that those who know nothing about dying know nothing about living either and they find it hard to discover a meaning in their lives. Perhaps if Amanda had initially come face-to-face with her fear of death, she would not have been so afraid to live and she would have been free of anxiety and IBS.

In this chapter, I have tried to explore the meaning of spiritual health and looked particularly at the extremes of life – old age and childhood. I have also touched on the importance of considering the spiritual dimension in mental illness and illustrated how this incorporation may be crucial to promoting healing in homeopathic medicine.

We might choose to consider the existence of the spiritual dimension or of the soul something insignificant. Many people believe otherwise. This belief colours their life experience and their approach to health, illness and suffering. It is evident in the patient narratives that follow in the next chapter. We cannot afford to ignore the spiritual dimension if we want to understand ourselves, others and the experience of health and illness. Others would agree:

'Just as a candle cannot burn without fire, men cannot live without a spiritual life.'

Buddha

'You have to grow from the inside out. None can teach you, none can make you spiritual. There is no other teacher but your own soul.'

Swami Vivekananda

REFERENCES

1 Caretta F, Petrini M. *Ai confine del dolore: salute e malattia nelle culture religiose*. Rome: Città Nuova; 1999 (author's translation).
2 Firshein J. Spirituality in medicine gains support in the USA. *Lancet*. 1997; **349**: 1300.
3 Levin JS. How religion influences morbidity and health: reflections on natural history, salutogenesis and host resistance. *Soc Sci Med*. 1996; **43**(5): 849–64.
4 Levin JS, Schiller PL. Is there a religious factor in health? *J Relig Health*. 1987; **26**: 9–36.
5 Jarvis JK, Northcutt HC. Religious differences in morbidity and mortality. *Soc Sci Med*. 1987; **25**: 813–24.
6 Smith T. *Homoeopathic Medicine for Mental Health*. Rochester: Healing Arts Press; 1989.
7 Morris T. *Philosophy for Dummies*. Hoboken: John Wiley & Sons; 1999.
8 Gledhill R. 'Psyche: show a little spirit'. *The Times*. 6 March 2004.
9 www.show.scot.nhs.uk
10 Hungelmann J, Kenkel-Rossi E, Klassen L, *et al*. Focus on spiritual well-being. *Geriatr Nurs*. 1996; **17**(6): 262–6.
11 Koenig HG, McCullough ME, Larson DB. *Handbook of Religion and Health*. New York: Oxford University Press; 2000.
12 Coleman PG, Mills M, McKiernan F, *et al*. Spiritual belief and quality of life: the experience of older bereaved spouses. *Qual Ageing Policy Practice Res*. 2002; **3**: 20–6.
13 American Psychiatric Association. *Diagnostic and Statistical Manual of Mental Disorders*. 4th ed. Washington, DC: American Psychiatric Association; 1994.
14 Davies R. www.quotationspage.com/quote/26290.html
15 Cicero MT. *Treatises on Friendship and Old Age*. Shuckburgh ES, translator. 1900.
16 Wordsworth W. *In Her Seventieth Year*. 1827.
17 Coulehan J. *The Knitted Glove*. Troy: Nightshade Press; 1991.
18 www.quotationspage.com/quote/8040.html
19 Barrett J. Born believers: the naturalness of childhood theism. Lecture given at the Faraday Institute, Cambridge University on 25 November 2008. Accessible at: www.st-edmunds.cam.ac.uk/faraday/Multimedia.php
20 Barnes LL, Plotnikoff GA, Fox K, *et al*. Subject reviews: spirituality, religion, and pediatrics; intersecting worlds of healing. *Pediatrics*. 2000; **106**(4) Supplement: 899–908.
21 Jessing B. Back to Square One. In: Haddad AM, Brown KH, editors. *The Arduous Touch: women's voices in healthcare*. West Lafayette: Notabell Books, Purdue University Press; 1999.
22 Coles R. *The Spiritual Life of Children*. Glasgow: HarperCollins; 1992.
23 Ryken L. *The Liberated Imagination: thinking christianly about the arts*. Wheaten: H Shaw Books; 1989.
24 Bridger F. *A Charmed Life: the spirituality of Potterworld*. London: Darton, Longman & Todd; 2001.
25 Fynn. *Anna and Mr God*. London: HarperCollins; 2004.

26 Zattoni M, Gillini G. *When Children Suffer Through Conflicts, Suffering & Loss*. Chawton: Many Rooms Publishing; 2002.

27 De Saint-Exupery A. *The Little Prince*. Woods K, translator. London: Puffin Books; 1973.

28 Koenig HG, Bearon LB, Dayringer R. Physician perspectives on the role of religion in the physician-older patient relationship. *J Fam Pract*. 1989; **28**: 441–8.

29 The Royal College of Psychiatrists. www.rcpsych.ac.uk/mentalhealthinformation/therapies/spiritualityandmentalhealth.aspx

30 Ionata P. *Psicoterapia e Problematiche Religiose: esperienze potenzialità e limit*. Rome: Città Nuova Editrice; 1993.

31 www.viktorfrankl.org/e/logotherapy.html

32 Ulz E. *L'uomo è l'artefice della sua vita* (Man is the architect of his life). Rome: Città Nuova; 2005.

33 Holmes OW. Homeopathy and its Kindred Delusions. Delivered before the Boston Society for the Diffusion of Useful Knowledge. 1842.

34 Grandgeorge D. *The Spirit of Homeopathic Medicines: essential insights into 300 remedies*. Berkeley: North Atlantic Books; 1998.

35 Ernst E, Pittler M, Wider B, *et al*. *Oxford Handbook of Complementary Medicine*. Oxford: OUP; 2008.

36 Barrett B, Marchand L, Scheder J, *et al*. What complementary and alternative medicine practitioners say about health and health care. *Ann Fam Med*. 2004; **2**(3): 253–9.

37 Hahnemann S. *Organon of Medicine*. Boericke WB, translator. New Delhi: B Jain; 2003.

38 Kent JT. *Lectures on Homeopathic Philosophy*. New Delhi: B Jain; 2003.

39 Vithoulkas G. *The Science of Homoeopathy*. London: Thorsons, HarperCollins; 1986.

40 Gray B. Thuja – the great masquerade. *Homeopathic Links*. 1995; **2**: 9–11.

41 Reilly DT, Taylor MA, McSharry C, *et al*. Is homoeopathy a placebo response? Controlled trial of homoeopathic potency with pollen in hay fever as a model. *Lancet*. 1986; **2**: 881–6.

42 Kleijnen J, Knipschild P, ter Riet G. Clinical trials of homoeopathy. *BMJ*. 1991; **302**: 316–23.

43 Clarke JH. *Dictionary of Practical Materia Medica*. 1900

44 Vithoulkas G. *The Essence of Materia Medica*. New Delhi: B Jain; 1993.

45 Amiri B, Wood B. *Some Cactaceae in Homeopathic Medicine. Notes from the 2005 – 11th Summer Seminar in Alghero by Dr Massimo Mangialavori*. Modena: Matrix Editrice; 2006.

46 Reilly D, Duncan R, Bikker AP, *et al*. Development of GHHOS, The IDCCIM Action Research & the PC-HICOM Project. Interim Report, February 2003. www.adhom.com/adh_download/PrimaryCarePrescribing.pdf

CHAPTER 4

Patient narratives

'Experience purchased by suffering teaches wisdom.'
Latin proverb

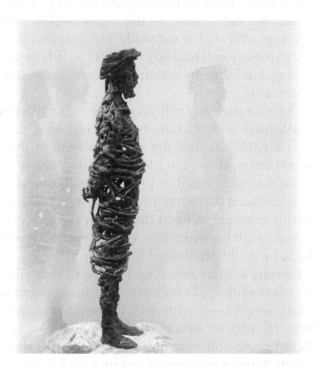

Survivor by Lau Hung

STORYTELLING

Changes in society – for example in postmodernist thought, social sciences, and cultural studies – have resulted in a revolution in thinking in diverse fields of learning. This revolution has led to a shift from the hitherto standard, accepted ways of understanding people to understanding through narrative. We are invited to see reality more like a 'tapestry of language that is continually being woven'.[1] This revolution is fired by an underlying concept: we construct our view of reality by telling our stories. As a result, particularly in mental healthcare, psychologists, psychotherapists and some psychiatrists have started to see their role more as facilitators in helping people to develop their stories about themselves. These health professionals are casting aside a top-down, authoritative view of patients and their illness. The idea here is that changing our stories, changes our view of reality. Listening to patients' stories also increases health professionals' understanding. Patient narratives are the 3-D glasses we need to view illness and illness experience.

For example, there is Gregor Samsa's story.[2] He wakes up one morning following a night of troubled dreams and finds himself strangely transformed into a 'monstrous cockroach'. No one seems able to explain why or how this has occurred. One thing is certain – it has happened and Gregor's metamorphosis appears to be irreversible. Gregor's first reaction is denial: 'What if I went back to sleep for a while, and forgot about all this nonsense?' He attempts to do so, but cannot even turn over on his right side. He feels revulsion at his metamorphosis as on trying to touch his body to relieve an itch he 'assayed the place with one of the legs, but hurriedly withdrew it, because the touch caused him to shudder involuntarily'.[2]

Gregor next looks for the cause of his condition and attributes it to his work as a travelling salesman with its long hours, bad meals, uncertainties and vicissitudes. It is a wild idea, but the only explanation that he can offer. Irrationally, he still attempts to get up from bed, thinking of getting the next train to work even though it would be physically nigh impossible. The denial continues. He has no doubt the change in his voice is just the first sign of a head cold. He eventually manages to open the door with his mouth. Despite his changed appearance with his many legs and the sticky substance emanating from his footpads, he is still determined to go to work.

Gregor has difficulty in communicating. He understands others but his voice is like 'the voice of an animal'. His father makes hissing noises while he drives him back into the room. It never occurs to his family that he can actually understand everything. He tries to reconnect with humanity – his own and the humanity of those around him – but now Gregor is seen as alien. He continues to lose touch with 'humanity'. Lying down in a high-ceilinged room is uncomfortable for him so with a half unconscious turn, and not without a little shame, he hurries under the sofa, where he straightaway feels very much at home, despite the confined space. He feels mortified by his body and wants to hide. Gregor now has a revulsion for fresh food but avidly eats the cheese that a couple of days before he had declared unfit for human consumption.

Initially his sister overcomes her disgust to attend to his basic needs with some care. He realises however that his appearance is unbearable to the whole family. Relations with his family deteriorate. His food is eventually kicked into the room and then hooked out in the evening with a broom. His room gets dirtier and more neglected. He becomes thinner, weaker and more ill.

One evening, Gregor's sister plays the violin for the tenants the family is forced to take in because of financial hardship. Unlike the insensitive tenants, Gregor is enthralled and asks himself if he could be an animal to be so moved by music.

The communication with his family breaks down so much that all of Gregor's good intentions are misunderstood. Rejection meets his attempts to draw closer. His sister's words resound painfully in his ear:

> I don't want to speak the name of my brother within the hearing of that monster, and so I will merely say: we have to try to get rid of it. We did as much as humanly possible to try and look after and tolerate it...If it was Gregor he would long ago have seen that it is impossible for human beings to live together with an animal like that, and he would have left of his own free will.

Gregor dies shortly after and the family, by now indifferent, are greeted by the chilling words of the insolent serving woman: '...it's gone and perished...you don't have to worry about how to get rid of the thing next door. I'll take care of it.'

Gregor's story is tragic and not unlike the story of people who in some way feel ostracised by others. People with chronic illness may feel different – perhaps alien. I wonder what went on inside Gregor. The author speaks of his physical and emotional problems. Did Gregor perhaps ask himself the meaning of his existence and the purpose of his life? Perhaps this question is implicit in the story itself.

Metamorphosis is, if you like, an elaborate patient narrative. Just simply describing the condition of 'instectametamorphosis' would read like a uni-dimensional case history:

> The pathology develops overnight and results in an appearance and behaviour similar to that of a cockroach. There is a total absence of human characteristics and the inability to communicate meaningfully. Weight loss and death follow without any return to the human state.

Gregor's story instead tells us how he coped with the condition and the meaning (or lack of meaning) ascribed to it.

If we took the time from our ever so busy schedules to listen to patients...they too would tell us stories of the metamorphosis which illness produces. For some this change is as awful and tragic as Gregor's. However, for others it is a prelude to something much more beautiful – the chrysalis before the butterfly emerges.

Stories may help us explore spirituality. Stephen Kliewer and John Saultz present different models of spirituality, which could be used as a framework to draw out spiritual experience from narratives.[3] One model looks at the six dimensions of spirituality proposed by Charles Ndlela.

1 The ideological dimension concerns a person's beliefs or values.
2 The intellectual dimension involves 'raw knowledge'.
3 The ritualistic dimension includes anything from formalised worship to creating a sacred space.
4 The experiential dimension is the presence of the divine or sacred: the sensation of connection to something greater than the self.
5 The consequential dimension shows the influence of spirituality on everyday activities.
6 The supportive dimension comprises social support and community participation.

Another model for exploring spirituality is to regard it as a journey or quest. The five phases of the journey involve:

1 the call to the journey because of disturbing uneasiness and dissatisfaction
2 crossing the threshold into the unknown
3 the trials and tribulations of the journey
4 attainment and enlightment
5 the return of the hero.[3]

PATIENT NARRATIVES

The best way to tell a story is to let the narrator use his or her own words. The following storytellers are people who simply volunteered to share their stories of how they cope with illness. From the interviews that follow, it appears that many of their resources are spiritual. The names of the patients are fictitious while 'D' refers to 'doctor'.

I think he is very nice and does his best to help you

The name Jennifer Cavilleri-Barrett will probably mean nothing to most people, but those who are familiar with 1970s films will know *Love Story*. Two young people from different social classes fall in love and marry. They have to struggle financially because the father of the rich young man angrily severs his connection. The young husband discovers that Jennifer has leukaemia – a condition that is almost a taboo subject. Sadly, she dies.

Leukaemia still evokes fear today – understandably so. It is a cancer of the white blood cells, which proliferate uncontrollably, and madly destroy normal tissue. Perhaps the frightening thing about leukaemia is its ability to strike the very young as well as the very old. The treatment seems to be almost as aggressive as the condition and results in hair loss, an even weaker immune system and mouth ulcers. Leukaemia therapy amounts to tough tactics and politicians have not been slow to seize the imagery it conjures:

> 'To cure the British disease with socialism was like trying to cure leukaemia with leeches.'
>
> Margaret Thatcher

Lucy is a young girl with leukaemia. She is bright and fun loving – an ordinary girl in every respect. This is her story.

D: You've got leukaemia. How long have you had that for and how was it discovered?

Lucy: I started to get really unusual bruises when I didn't knock.... I had a lot of pains in my legs and was tired a lot and every time I picked up a cold, I couldn't get rid of it.

D: Had you ever heard of the word 'leukaemia' before?

Lucy: On telly, but that was it.

D: So what idea did you have of the word 'leukaemia'?

Lucy: Mmm...really I just thought that it was something wrong with the blood.

D: Did you think anything more about it?

Lucy: I knew you lost your hair. And you didn't always die from it. When they told me that I did have it, I knew that there was a good chance for me to come through it.

D: When you were told, were you frightened?

Lucy: Yes, mainly because I thought I was going to lose my hair.

D: And you lost your hair?

Lucy: I lost all of it...I didn't even have stubble. It was just bald.

D: How did you feel about that?

Lucy: Well, at first, that was what upset me the most. And when we knew my transplant was coming up, we got it cut short...so that when the time came for losing it, I didn't feel that I had lost as much because I got it cut short, so I was OK with it then.

D: When you lost it, were you very upset?

Lucy: Yes...I only lost it once...after my transplant. It kept on falling off and irritating me, so we had to shave it off.

D: Did you ever have any pain – from anything?

Lucy: I had a lot of pain after the radiation because of blisters inside my mouth and all down my throat...and a lot of gut pain where it had all burned but...and my legs...

D: And did that upset you a lot?

Lucy: The main thing that upset me really was my mouth. I couldn't eat at all.

D: So how did you manage?

Lucy: Basically it was my mum and dad telling me that if I do this it will get better. We had a lot of mouth care to do, and sometimes I just felt too sick to do it but my parents were always saying to me 'if you do it, it will get better' and even though I felt sick I would do it and then it was only about a week and it got better...

D: OK, you're only twelve years old and you've had to go through quite a lot of things and who knows what you're going to have to go through in the future. Another person who is twelve years old or even someone who is older could ask themselves, 'But how did you manage to cope with all this?'

Lucy: Basically because I didn't want to die, I just didn't want to die. I just said to myself in my head 'you've got to get through this' – and prayers.

D: Who prayed for you?

Lucy: I prayed a lot myself, my mum, my dad and all my family. I had masses said for me and stuff like that.

D: So, prayers are very important for you?

Lucy: Yes.

D: So if you pray, do you believe in God?

Lucy: Yes.

D: What do you imagine? What do you think God is like?

Lucy: I think he is very nice and does his best to help you. He is always with you and sometimes there are just things he can't control.

D: So do you think he is always with you?

Lucy: Yes.

D: Does that make you feel better?

Lucy: Yes.

D: Do you think he sees everything?

Lucy: Yes.

D: When you say there are things he can't control, what sort of things can't he control?

Lucy: Like, emm, he can't always control who gets it and who doesn't.

D: So you think that is outside his control and yet you say he loves you?

Lucy: Yes.

D: Do you think he loves you very much?

Lucy: Yes. He loves everybody very much.

D: Do you think so, Lucy, but someone could say, 'If God loves you very much, how come you've got this condition? What would you say to them?'

Lucy: I'd say that he loves everybody, but he just can't help it. It is nothing to do with him. It's something in your body.

D: Right...but you think that he loves you and he helps you.

Lucy: Yes.

D: Do you think that having the illness has made you a braver person?

Lucy: Yes.

D: So, it has changed you?

Lucy: Oh yes!!!

D: So what other thing has it made you that you wouldn't have been before, do you think, without this illness?

Lucy: Well now, instead of worrying about things I should worry about, I worry about things that I didn't. I get a sore leg and I think all kinds of things and stuff.

D: Because you know what it could be in other words. Do you think it has helped you understand people better?

Lucy: Yes.

D: In what way?

Lucy: I think it just makes you realise that no matter what people have got and how their appearance has changed, don't criticise them or nothing like that because it's not their fault and you know that they can't control it.

D: Do you think you can put up with people more?

Lucy: Yes.

D: Now, Lucy, I'm going to ask you a hard question. You say that God loves you, but have you ever felt angry with him because of what you've got? Ever?

Lucy: No.

D: Have you ever felt angry with anyone?

Lucy: Yes, my mum, dad, brothers and sisters.

D: Why is that? Or do you not want to talk about it?

Lucy: I don't know. Sometimes I can just get angry with everyone: 'you don't love me any more' and stuff like that. I don't know why I get angry. I just get these sudden urges and want to throw things at people and stuff like that.

D: Is that when you are feeling really ill?

Lucy: No. It just happens every now and again and I get bad-tempered and stuff but when I feel ill I always want my mum and dad and everyone around me.

D: Now you said before, Lucy, that you said to yourself, 'I want to live! I want to live!' We all die don't we? I'm going to die. We all die eventually. What do you think happens to us after we die?

Lucy: Emm.

D: Do you know anyone that has died?

Lucy: Yes, my grandparents.

D: Where do you think they are now?

Lucy: In heaven.

D: So you believe that there is a heaven. You believe that we'll all go there?

Lucy: Well, there are stages and some people might never get to the top one.

D: Yes...and tell me about those stages? How do you see these stages?

Lucy: I dunno...like clouds really.

D: And what are they like – these clouds?

Lucy: I dunno...just clouds...and people on them.

D: And do you think we have to go from one stage to the other, like, to go up higher and higher?

Lucy: I think you've got to sort of earn it.

D: And how do you think you earn it?

Lucy: Just by watching over the people you love and stuff like that.

D: So you feel that you've got to be giving, that you've got to be loving to other people and then you go from one stage to the other. What stage do you think you're at?

Lucy: Well, I don't know about that.

D: But you think you've got to earn it?

Lucy: Yes.

D: Do you think that is what we have got to do in our life? To try to 'earn' it?

Lucy: I don't know.

D: Would you think that your illness is part of earning it when you have moments when it is difficult or when you've got the treatment to get or have you not thought of it in that way?

Lucy: No...not really.

D: It's just one of those things and you get on with your life.

Lucy: Yes.

If I didn't believe in God...I probably couldn't be bothered

Cystic fibrosis (CF) is one of the commonest genetic conditions in the Caucasian population of the UK. It affects 1 in every 2500 infants. Typically, parents may bring their child to see the GP because 'Jimmy keeps getting one infection after the other', or 'Keira does not seem to be putting on as much weight as her siblings did at her age'. The child's lungs are normal at birth but become diseased. Cystic fibrosis sufferers have a productive, tormenting cough.

Diane Gilliam Fisher writes movingly in her poetry about living with her daughter's CF. Like many parents she had never heard of CF but she had noticed the saltiness of her daughter's skin whenever she kissed her.

Elsewhere Fisher poignantly describes how a little boy with the condition, misunderstanding its name, would tell his classmates that he could not breathe properly because he had 'sixty-five roses' in his chest.[4] In another poem, Fisher paints a domestic picture of her now 16-year-old daughter's coughing fits in between the 'crescendo, decrescendo' of her violin playing. The coughing bouts last ten to fifteen minutes and the author holds her breath each time she stops.[5]

Like Fisher's daughter, 14-year-old Anna has cystic fibrosis and this is her story.

D: When did you first become aware that you sometimes weren't well?

Anna: I don't know. I've just always done my physio and stuff.

D: Have you ever found it hard to do your physio because I'm sure it must be a bit of a nuisance at times?

Anna: Yes. In year five and six, about four-and-a-half years ago...

D: How old would you have been at the time...nine or ten?

Anna: Maybe a bit younger. I got a bit sick of doing it. I still did it, it's just that...

D: Anna – you know the times when you say that you don't feel like doing it – what helps you go ahead to do it? What helps you carry on with it?

Anna: I just know that if I don't do it, I get really ill and I'll just cough more during the day. I don't know really, it's just habit. I just know that I have to do it.

D: Would you say that sometimes your belief in God makes a difference?

Anna: Sometimes.

D: When would you say that it makes a difference to you?

Anna: Not in doing anything but just in knowing that I've got CF but it doesn't really matter 'cos I'm supposed to. Do you know what I mean?

D: So you mean in the sense that you've got CF, God knows that you've got CF and he'll give you the strength to live with the CF. Do you mean it in that way? What importance does God have for you?

Anna: Well, everything I do, I try to do what is best...I don't know. He is just important. Like...if I do something, like trying to do it right for God.

D: So, he's very important to you.

Anna: Yes.

D: God is very important to you in your life and he gives a lot of meaning to the things that you do, be it to the cystic fibrosis, but not just that...be it to the things that you do every day.

Anna: Yes.

D: And if God wasn't there – let's put it this way – all the things that you do or even the fact that you've got cystic fibrosis, wouldn't have so much meaning. Is that right?

Anna: Yes.

D: Fine. Have I understood properly?

Anna: Yes. You know I go to hospital for a check up and things? Well I went on a ski trip with them, with all the people who have CF. One of the girls who was about my age, we had similar interests and things, she was like trying not to admit that she had CF. She was pretending...like she doesn't want to have any connection to the hospital when she has to go. That means that she doesn't do half her treatments and things and when she gets ill she has to go into hospital. If I didn't believe in God and that this is right, I probably couldn't be bothered and wouldn't see the point in it like that...

I must have a good spirit

Munch's painting *The Scream* is a potent symbol of psychic agony. It could however also represent physical agony, torment and torture from which there does not seem to be any escape. Munch describes the sensations, which he associates with the picture:

> I stood there trembling with fright and I felt a loud, unending scream piercing nature.

Screaming is what Molly has often found herself doing. She suffers from intractable, chronic pain. The pain is due to neuralgia following an attack of Herpes zoster (shingles). Such pain may persist for several months, but in Molly's case, it has plagued her for several years.

D: How old are you?
Molly: I'm 86.
D: And you've had very bad pain since you had shingles 15 years ago?
Molly: Well this is different entirely to the shingles pain but I've learned to live with that. It's like electric shocks and I have to grab hold of somebody. It can happen many times and it wakes me up from sleep. There is no pattern to it. I might be in the middle of Marks and Spencer and everyone came running they thought it was a heart attack. My husband kept saying, 'She's alright!'
D: How long does it last for when it comes?
Molly: Well that depends. Sometimes it's very sharp and short. Other times it will go on and on I would say for ten spasms. And even when it's finished, it's just like a little wriggling, red hot wire going through. It's most unusual.
D: I see a large variety of people and I'm always interested in knowing about how they live with the conditions that they've got. What resources they have...
Molly: I agree!
D: ...to cope with them. You try to help as much as you can with medicines but then some people seem to have more inner resources than others. What would you say helps you?
Molly: Well, years ago I would have agreed with you when I had the rheumatoid arthritis pretty bad. That is when I was on the steroids. I sort of accepted that and I was alright but I started getting all kinds of odd things. I went into hospital with a suspected heart attack and came out with gallstones, a duodenal ulcer and a hiatus hernia. I've learned to live with all that.
D: How did you learn to live with those things?
Molly: I think that people got fed up of listening to me moaning. My husband helped a lot because he has got the patience of a saint. But then again not everyone is lucky like me...I sort of put a brave face on things. I remember the doctor saying all those years ago that rheumatoid arthritis can burn itself out. On top of all that, I've got osteoporosis of my spine and in my back three vertebrae have crumbled away so I'm on medication for that. And then I've had a stroke and since the stroke I think I've lost a bit of heart.

D: What makes you say that?

Molly: Well, I'm getting depressed. When I first came out of the hospital I never stopped crying for two days and I had to send for the doctor and he explained that it was the effect of the stroke. Friends will come round and say 'I hope I look as good as you at your age' but looks don't mean anything! You feel like something the cat dragged in. And then I think they don't know, they don't understand. And now, of course I'm older now, aren't I? But you can't cope with things the same, can you?

D: I don't know. I know that things are harder as you get older. The health that can buck you up and that we take for granted isn't there anymore and everything is more of an effort...

Molly: I think getting into the wheelchair didn't help. I won't go in that wheelchair at all outside the door...I mean the car was going then and he would just put the wheelchair in the boot and we would go anywhere.

D: And why won't you get in the wheelchair now?

Molly: I'm in it all the time.

D: But you wouldn't go outside? Why not?

Molly: Because people know me and I don't want them stopping me and asking me how I am.

D: Have you accepted having had the stroke and the pain you've got from the shingles?

Molly: Well, that's a very hard thing to say with the stroke. Thank God, this one isn't nearly as bad as the first one. The first one I was dead all down one side like a piece of wood. This time I wasn't like that. In fact a funny thing happened. I found I started to use my right hand after the second one. So it was a blessing in disguise.

D: So where had the first stroke been. Did it affect the right side?

Molly: Yes.

D: So are you using your right hand more since you had the second stroke?

Molly: Yes. I can use a knife and fork. My thumb has never been much use to me.

D: Can you give any sort of meaning to having had the stroke or the pain?

Molly: Except that I must have been awfully wicked when I was a child because they say that only the good die young and I'm still here.

D: Do you seriously believe that though?

Molly: No! It's just been one of those things and I've been unfortunate. I've had this breathing business since I was in my teens, so you learn to live with it. You take no notice of it in the end unless something like this happens.

D: Has it altered you as a person?

Molly: No.

D: In the sense of the way you react to other people?

Molly: I'm still as popular. I have marvellous, wonderful friends.

D: Has it helped you appreciate things in other people that you maybe hadn't appreciated in them before? Has it changed your outlook in any way?

Molly: I don't think so. It may have done but I haven't noticed.

D: We all give different meanings to what we experience...

Molly: I would say that the older you get, the easier it is to accept it. You take it for granted that it's age – well I do. Because I've been very, very lively. I've never walked anywhere. I've always run.

D: Do you try to give any sort of spiritual meaning to the pain or to the illnesses that you've had?

Molly: Well, that's hard, because I'm very fond of prayer. I pray quite a bit. The trouble is that I pray of a night time when I can't go to sleep. Does that make sense?

D: Yes, it does.

Molly: I pray for those who have gone. I start praying for those who are in trouble.

D: Does your pain relate in any way to the fact that you've had a stroke or to the pain from the shingles?

Molly: To be honest, the stroke has only happened this year and I've had the pain of the shingles for years.

D: Well, let's talk about the pain of the shingles. How do you explain that in terms of your spiritual beliefs or can't you explain it? You believe in God...?

Molly: Oh yes. I'm a RC [Roman Catholic] and I'm very much into prayer.

D: Has your prayer life and your faith helped you to accept your condition?

Molly: I don't think so. I'm not consciously aware of it.

D: Let's say, if I were to take away your prayer life...do you think you would be able to give your condition any meaning or would you be able to accept it just as well, do you think?

Molly: I don't think that I could do that.

D: Why not?

Molly: Faith I suppose.

D: But why could you not live without it?

Molly: I've no idea. It's just a feeling I've got.

D: Do you think it's a feeling that gives some sort of meaning or purpose to what you go or live through?

Molly: That may be so. I've haven't thought of that but I can see the point.

D: Do you believe in an afterlife?

Molly: Yes.

D: Do you feel that a lot of what you suffer here has got something to do with what you're going to live after?

Molly: Now, they always say, don't they, that if you're suffering on earth, you're paying for somebody's sins. Have you heard that?

D: I've heard of it...yes.

Molly: Well that's my philosophy. I've sort of accepted all this over the years. And I'm always cheerful – not like this – when people do come in. We'll have a good laugh and a good joke and they say, 'I don't know how you keep your spirits up.'

D: But do you ever feel any anger or resentment?

Molly: I do.

D: Who do you feel angry at?

Molly: I say, 'Why me?'

D: So who do you direct this anger at? Who to? Do you feel angry with God?

Molly: No!

D: Angry with yourself?

Molly: Well, that's a point I've never thought of. But I do resent having it all. Dr X says to me, 'But what else can go wrong? What are we going to do with her? What else can she get?'

D: But what makes you cheerful?

Molly: I don't know. My spirit, I suppose. Well, I must have a good spirit.

D: And what gives you this good spirit?

Molly: I don't know.

D: Do you know you've inspired me? Because I came to visit you after you had that stroke and I was really impressed at the way you seemed–

Molly: I accepted it.

D: Because I've seen people with strokes before and I've seen people of different ages with stroke...

Molly: Well I was lucky, wasn't I? Thank God for that. I didn't lose my speech. My face didn't twist up. I was very, very fortunate.

D: So you thanked God because you were aware of other things that could have gone wrong?

Molly: It could have been so much worse. No, I saw some of the patients at that stroke unit.

D: Can you walk at all?

Molly: No. I'll walk with my stick as far as the toilet.

D: A friend of mine has just had a stroke. What advice would you give her? What would you say to her?

Molly: Well, it wouldn't be advice as such. I would give her a bit of encouragement. I would say to her, 'Well it could have been a lot worse. That's my thanks to God – that it wasn't as bad as it could have been. The only thing is, this is my second one. And the doctor said, 'Two strokes in eight months: that sounds serious...'

Every day is a bonus to me

Laryngeal cancer (commonly known as throat cancer) affects 1 in 100,000 people. The classical case is an older man presenting to the GP with a history of persistent hoarseness. If the disease is detected early, the prognosis is good with 90% of patients surviving after 5 years. Many patients may present at a later stage, so the cure rate falls. The treatment may be quite devastating and involve radiotherapy and/or removal of the vocal cords. Patients have to learn how to speak using the oesophagus and to breathe through a hole in the throat (tracheotomy).

Abba Kovner was a Jew who fought against the Nazis during the Second World War in Lithuania. His wartime struggles against this aggression are mirrored in the poems of *Sloan Kettering*,[6] a collection describing his experience with laryngeal cancer. In a voiceless conversation, he speaks of his throat being 'in ruins' after surgery and elsewhere of the 'wreckage of his voice'.

Although laryngeal cancer is more common in men, Margaret also suffers from the condition.

D: People come to see me for five or ten minutes but often, I maybe don't fully appreciate how they try to live with what they've got in everyday life... I'm looking more from the aspect of the resources for coping that people have inside them because often what you feel inside drives what you do outside, I don't know if you would agree with that.
Margaret: Yes, I would.
D: So you've got cancer of the larynx and that was diagnosed how long ago?
Margaret: Before last Christmas.
D: So that was only about 16 months ago? What was it for you to know that diagnosis? Were you frightened by it?
Margaret: I was frightened at first. When he said the word 'cancer'.
D: What did it make you think of?
Margaret: I saw these people with holes in the throat when I went to the hospital and I thought thank God I am not like that...I have a great faith in God you know.
D: Has that faith in God been important for you all your life? Has it been important for you over the last 16 months?
Margaret: Yes.
D: In what way?
Margaret: Well I pray for my mother, father, brother...all the souls in purgatory.[†] Every night I say my prayers before I go to sleep.
D: You've lived with this over the last 16 months or so. In what way did your faith help you?

[†] The idea of purgatory has its origins in the religions of the ancient Middle East with special reference to Jewish and Christian Scriptures. During late antiquity and the Middle Ages, it was seen particularly as a condition or place of spiritual cleansing for the expiation of sins. Dante's epic poem 'La Divina Commedia' (Divine Comedy) was written during that time. It concerns the journey through hell, purgatory and paradise.

Margaret: Well I just prayed and put my faith in God. If he wants me, he'll take me. If he wants to cure me, he'll cure me.

D: So when you say you put your faith in God...

Margaret: My mother used to say, you can't fly in the face of God.

D: So when you say you put your faith in God, you mean you trusted in God?

Margaret: I do. You can't get along without the doctors, you know – with a little help from up above I think you can fight through some things.

D: So when you say this faith in God, did you not feel angry then with God?

Margaret: No.

D: You didn't feel angry with God at all?

Margaret: No, because I've had a good life. A lot of things happened.

D: How old are you by the way?

Margaret: Sixty-seven. I've had a really rough time.

[Margaret then describes some of her encounters with bereavement, pain and hardship.]

D: So how do you link all these past events and what you live now?

Margaret: Well, I don't know how I got the strength to do all this: I was green. I had to get by. I had no help from anyone. I had to get by on my own with my brothers and my sisters.

D: So you are telling me that because of what you went through, you've got the strength to go through anything.

Margaret: I've got the strength to go through anything else.

D: Do you think that what you went through before – that your faith helped you go through with that?

Margaret: Yes, I do.

D: What makes you think that?

Margaret: My mother had faith and we always went to church. We never missed church once...

D: Are you saying to me the fact that you knew that God existed helped you to carry on?

Margaret: I do.

D: What if you hadn't had a faith – how do you think that you would have managed?

[Here Margaret describes how the premature death of her brother resulted in a deep spiritual crisis.]

Margaret: Well, that was a knock and I questioned God then. And then I said to myself, 'why should I question him? Maybe it's for the best because he separated from his wife'...he neglected himself in every way and that's why I looked after him when he came back. I made sure he got a dinner and break-fast. That is the only time that I have lost faith. And then when my husband died he would have had to have his legs cut off and that would have killed him anyway, so that was a blessing in disguise because he would never have lived with it. So I've suffered. I really have. Because I've lived and loved everyone. Well I'm happy now for my son. As long as God keeps him safe, I don't mind – and my brother and sisters.

D: When you say that you've suffered, what have you learnt from the experience of suffering?

Margaret: Well, I've learned to listen to people and there is always somebody worse off than me. That's why I don't annoy the doctors. I try not to. I would be dying here and I just wouldn't call them [the doctors] out. I think that in all the years that I've been here, I think that I've had them out about five times and I've been on the books for many years.

D: When you say that suffering has taught you to listen, is it not something that you would have learned anyway without suffering?

Margaret: I don't know. No...you don't know about death until you go through it. People say, 'Oh yes! I know how you feel.' But nobody knows how you feel when you lose your mother, your father, your brother, your husband. Nobody knows how you feel. You can be laughing and joking but inside there is a knot there. Even today, I think of them all. I think of the happy times we had and it's a comfort.

D: Would you say that the experience that you have gone through...

Margaret: ...Has made me stronger.

D: Would you say that?

Margaret: Yes!

D: Would you say that it has enriched you as a person? Enriched in the sense that it's made you understand other people?

Margaret: I cannot understand people being selfish. That's one thing I don't like. And I don't like backbiters. You know people say, 'She's always the same...she's always the same. You hear it in that post office when you go down...'

D: If I were to take you to someone who has just been diagnosed with cancer, what would you say to him?

Margaret: Well, I would say, 'It's a terrible thing. It's something you can't help. So all you have to do is to try and face it. You should think back on the good times you've had and think of the family and friends that love you and who'll be there for you.' When you think of these poor people with AIDs. Well, that's a different thing entirely from cancer. I don't think that I would know what to say to them – especially young fellas of 23. It breaks my heart just looking at them. The sorrow would be there for them. I mean I've had a good life. I'm 67...you know it's a bonus. Every day is a bonus to me. That's what my husband used to say. Every day is a bonus when he was diagnosed with his legs.

D: And do you think that if a young person was in that situation, that if he had faith it would make a difference to him?

Margaret: Yes I do. You get a contentment. Even when I go into church now...and the peace that comes on you is lovely. You know, if you are worried about anything you just go in and sit down and say a few prayers and it's lovely. It really is...the contentment that fills you.

D: Do you think that the way we feel inside, our relationship with God or whatever we believe in has some relationship with the way that we feel physically?

Margaret: Yes.

D: What relationship do you think that is?

Margaret: He gives me comfort. If I pray every night I go to sleep right away and I feel comforted.

D: And that makes you feel physically better?

Margaret: I'm able to get up the next morning. Some nights I go to bed and I think that I don't want to get up. I get up and I do my day's work and I say, 'Thank God!'

D: And he gives you something to live for...

Margaret: ...Something to live for. Well, he's given me something; he's given me David [her son]. He's who I am living for now.

D: And if I had to ask you to just say in a few words what meaning having this illness has had for you, what would you say? What meaning has it got for you?

Margaret: Well, doctor, I try to think of what I've done really wrong in my life to be quite truthful. But as I say, as God closes one door, he always opens another. That's the only way that I can look at it. I haven't done any wrong. I've done no wrong to anyone. All I've wanted is my home.

D: So what door has God closed for you, would you say?

Margaret: My taste.

D: And what door has he opened for you?

Margaret: That I'm still living and I haven't got a hole in my throat. I could be worse, you know. I could have cancer right through my body. I could have a hole in my throat like that poor man. I was sick when I saw him. I've never seen anyone before like that. And yet they were lovely when I got to know them. I couldn't look at it. You know, when they were speaking to me. I just couldn't look at it because I kept thinking, 'Oh God! Don't ever let me go like that!' Have you seen it?

D: A tracheotomy. ..

Margaret: And he was only young, you know. He was only about 40.

D: How do you think he coped with it?

Margaret: I saw him when I went up about two months ago and he waved to me and I waved to him and I went over to him and he said to me, 'Are you alright?' And I said to him, 'But I still haven't got my taste back.' And he said. 'It will come back. It will come back.'

D: What made him cope with that condition?

Margaret: I don't know. You see, maybe he had inner strength. It might be his religion. Different people cope in different ways. I mean you hear in the papers, 'So and so has got cancer', but they ought to think of poor people who've got cancer and haven't got the money to spare for treatment like they've got the money to spare for their business and private homes. I thank God that I've got you and the other doctors. I know I can go to them. But think of the other poor people. I've been pretty lucky. They've looked after me pretty well.

Once you've done what you're supposed to have done, then that's it

Lucy, Anna, Molly and Margaret have all met their illnesses head on and in their daily struggles try to find meaning in their suffering. They have described how the spiritual dimension of their health affects how they manage their illness and vice versa. The importance to them of their spirituality emerged during the interviews. It was clear that despite – or because of – their pain, illness resulted in spiritual growth.

John Milton ranks second only to Shakespeare among English poets.[7] In 1652 at the age of 43, he went completely blind following years of visual problems. He wrote this poem about his blindness:

> **On His Blindness**
> When I consider how my light is spent
> Ere half my days in this dark world and wide,
> And that one Talent which is death to hide
> Lodged with me useless, though my soul more bent
> To serve therewith my Maker, and present
> My true account, lest He returning chide,
> 'Doth God exact day-labour, light denied?'
> I fondly ask. But Patience, to prevent
> That murmur, soon replies, 'God doth not need
> Either man's work or his own gifts. Who best
> Bear his mild yoke, they serve him best. His state
> Is kingly: thousands at his bidding speed,
> And post o'er land and ocean without rest;
> They also serve who only stand and wait.

A few years after he went blind, he wrote the epic poem 'Paradise Lost'.

Not everyone of course feels any sense of spiritual growth through illness even though all – whether religious or not – may experience a spiritual crisis. Beethoven's deafness was a hard, bitter trial for him. He could not bring himself to admit publically that he had this disability, particularly to his rivals:

Alas! how could I proclaim the deficiency of a sense which ought to have been more perfect with me than with other men, – a sense which I once possessed in the highest perfection, to an extent, indeed, that few of my profession ever enjoyed! Alas, I cannot do this! ... But what humiliation when any one beside me heard a flute in the far distance, while I heard *nothing*, or when others heard *a shepherd singing*, and I still heard *nothing*! Such things brought me to the verge of desperation, and well nigh caused me to put an end to my life. *Art! art* alone, deterred me. Ah! ... Perhaps I may get better, perhaps not. I am prepared for either. Constrained to become a philosopher in my twenty-eighth year! This is no slight trial, and more severe on an artist than on any one else...[8]

Heiligenstadt, 6 October 1802,
from a letter to brothers Carl and Johann

Fearing that his deafness might be exposed, he shunned the company of others who misunderstood him as this testament shows:

Oh! ye who think or declare me to be hostile, morose, and misanthropical, how unjust you are, and how little you know the secret cause of what appears thus to you! My heart and mind were ever from childhood prone to the most tender feelings of affection, and I was always disposed to accomplish something great. But you must remember that six years ago I was attacked by an incurable malady, aggravated by unskilful physicians, deluded from year to year, too, by the hope of relief, and at length forced to the conviction of a *lasting affliction*...[8]

Suicide tempted him but Art alone deterred him: 'How could I possibly quit the world before bringing forth all that I felt it was my vocation to produce?'

In 1802 when Beethoven went completely deaf, his life changed direction. He could no longer perform as a virtuoso, so he concentrated on composing. The irony is that much of his important music was composed in the last ten years of his life when he was completely deaf.

If disease does not respect talent or even genius, neither does it regard beauty, wealth or celebrity status. Jackie Onassis Kennedy suffered from non-Hodgkin's lymphoma in common with Linda, a young mum. Lymphoma is a tumour involving the lymph glands. Patients often present to their doctor with swollen glands, ignorant that they have a serious condition.

This is Linda's story.

D: So you've got lymphoma. How long have you had it?
Linda: About 5 years. My glands were a bit swollen and the doctor tested it. They found out it was a tumour. I didn't feel ill or anything.
D: So it all came quite suddenly, really. Were you quite shocked?
Linda: I felt alarmed...

D: How did they actually tell you? When did you start to feel alarmed?

Linda: I think it was when I started having treatment and I was losing my hair. Because I felt fine up to then. I was having injections. It was just this vomiting and...

D: So it wasn't the illness in itself. It was just the side effects of the treatment that they gave you. And when they told you that it was non Hodgkin's lymphoma, what did it mean to you?

Linda: I didn't really think about it. I don't think it's really sunk in. I just take everything as it comes.

D: Do you know anyone who has had lymphoma or you've never met anyone?

Linda: A few people in the hospital I've spoken to.

D: And how much have you been able to learn about the condition?

Linda: Not much really. As I say, I don't really think about it that much. I don't like to talk about it. It's just an everyday thing. It is just there.

[Some months before and after the diagnosis, Linda's sister and partner died.]

D: So you've had an awful lot on your plate. How have you been able to cope with all this?

Linda: I look at my children.

D: What sort of relationship do you have with them?

Linda: They know everything. I go to hospital and I tell them everything. What's going on. They got told about three years ago when I had steroids...I keep going.

D: So you're a fighter.

Linda: Oh yeah. You've got to be.

D: What makes you a fighter then?

Linda: My children. They are my life for me. I've always said that if I didn't have my children, I would be with Bill and Megan [partner and sister]. There would be nothing to fight for. I get up every morning and look at them, and I've got to [fight]. The little one doesn't really understand but me and the older one are really close. She knows when something is going on in my mind and when I'm upset. She had a couple of days off last week because she was complaining that she had tummy pain but I think she was worried about me...So every time I get ill, her poor little mind must be playing... 'This is it – mum is going straight away.'

D: Have you ever felt any anger or resentment at all?

Linda: Oh yeah – why me? What have I ever done? Bill used to say 'Why you? Of all people, you've never done anything.' I used to go to church, but now I can't bring myself to go to church.

D: So, when you say you used to go to church, you believed in God?

Linda: Yeah.

D: Where you baptised a Christian?

Linda: No, not really. I used to go but not every Sunday. I used to go and pray and that but then I lost Bill and Megan and I was ill and I thought, 'There can't be anyone there. No one is listening to me at the moment.'

D: Before all of this happened did you get comfort when you went to church?

Linda: Yes.

D: Like when you went to church, you obviously prayed and everything. Who did you pray to?

Linda: I don't know...I just felt...well the people were really nice and they were really friendly. I think that's what it was. I mean, I'm still on the sick list in the church.

D: When you were diagnosed with the lymphoma you still went to church.

Linda: For a while...

D: When did you stop going?

Linda: When I lost Bill.

D: Was that the final straw for you?

Linda: I think it was. I was so angry that I had to blame somebody, so I blamed God. [laughs] If there was someone.

D: Because you could take it as far as your illness up to a certain point, Megan's loss up to a certain point...

Linda: Well Megan was ill anyway.

D: But the loss of Bill seemed like a double blow.

Linda: It was the last straw: 'why me?'

D: Do you still get angry?

Linda: Yes.

D: When do you tend to get angry?

Linda: When I'm ill. I get frustrated.

D: Do you still get angry with God?

Linda: Not really.

D: So before you used to believe in the existence of Someone and now you don't believe. What do you believe in?

Linda: I don't know really. There must be Something...myself really. It's only me that can make myself better.

D: So the courage and everything you get is from looking at your children. When you look at your children, what do you see there?

Linda: All I hope, all I want, is to see them grown up. To see them possibly in a good job. I mean that's all I want. All I want is to see my children grow up. There is only me to watch them so it's all I ever wanted.

D: The fact that you know that people are praying for you does that make any difference?

Linda: Not really, no.

D: In other words – obviously we all like people to think of us – but if they stopped specifically praying for you...

Linda: It wouldn't bother me.

D: What sort of things – if anything – would you say you have learned from your experience of having lymphoma?

Linda: Take every day as it comes.

D: When you say, 'take every day as it comes' did you not do that before anyway or are you doing it in a different way now?

Linda: I've seen a lot of people in the hospital and I would have given up. A lot of my friends have died that I've got really close to. It's different. I take more time with the children and we have more holidays. I do as much as I can whereas before you just took it more for granted. I have more time to sit and listen to the children.

D: Has it made you value the time that you give to them more?

Linda: Yes, I think so. I don't know how much time I've got with them...

D: What other things have you learned to value more?

Linda: I don't know really. Take every day as it comes. You don't take things for granted. I don't plan ahead – that's one thing – and I don't make promises to the children. I'll say, 'We'll see how mummy is.' I don't know when I'm going to take ill again.

D: Would you not say that it's shown you that time is really precious? Suddenly things that you thought were important aren't so important anymore. Would you not say that this is something you've gained?

Linda: I think so; yes...nobody has given me a reason why I'm ill. If someone could sit down and tell me...it's just come. All I know is that it's in everybody, the cancer cells and everything and some people are just unfortunate.

D: How do you think that your children have grown up differently? What difference is there in them?

Linda: I think they are stronger...I seem to be closer to my parents since I've been ill. I'm sort of their little girl again...but illness can push people away as well. I've lost contact with the so-called friends that I thought I had. I think that they can't cope.

D: What can they not cope with?

Linda: I think it's the illness really. When I was having treatment I was really bad-tempered. I did change at one time...I can admit it...I can be really nasty. I think some of them can't cope.

D: Do you not think that they're afraid? They're the same age as you.

Linda: Yes, maybe...

D: They could think...

Linda: 'That could be me'...That's it maybe. Because when I was ill, they didn't know what to say or they would treat me differently.

D: In what way would they treat you differently?

Linda: Like with kid gloves...and it annoyed me. I said all along that I do not want sympathy. I just want to get on – you've got to. They say, 'How do you cope with it?' I've got to. I've seen it happen in the hospital. Once it kicks in and it takes over, you go under... You've got to fight for yourself.

D: Have you surprised yourself at how well you've coped?

Linda: Yes. I used to be a really weak person...but it has made me stronger. It's made me more forward as well. I'll speak to people now. At one time I was really shy and I would sort of cower in a corner but I'm really forward now. I'll go out and speak to people.

D: So would you not say that in a way there are two effects of an illness? There is the effect that it wears you down and everything but there have been a lot of things that have surprised you. What else has surprised you?

Linda: I've found out who my true friends are. My really close friends have stuck by me and my family.

D: What is your outlook in life? What would be the meaning of life for you? What do you think we're all here for?

Linda: I've never really thought about it. Well...we're all here for one purpose and once your purpose is done, your time is up.

D: So what purpose do you think we're here for? Who do you think decides that purpose?

Linda: Somebody.

D: So do you think that Somebody decides what purpose we live for and once we've fulfilled that purpose, that is the time for us to go?

Linda: [echoes] that is the time for us to go...

D: And do you think that Somebody decides the purpose of life for everyone?

Linda: I think so...it's like you're living through a play. You're put on this earth and once you've done what you're supposed to have done, then that's it.

D: Do you believe in an afterlife?

Linda: I don't know. I know my little girl says she has spoken to her dad. I'm not sure really. I would like to think that Bill and Megan are watching me.

D: So, if you believe that we all have a purpose in life, do you think that the suffering and pain that we go through has a purpose or do you think that it's just something that went wrong in the play?

Linda: It's just something that has happened, isn't it? It's just one of those things. You just get on with your life and try to fulfil the purpose that we're here for.

When I am at my 'illest', when I have least, my spirituality is stronger

The shrine of Our Lady of Lourdes is well-known not just to Catholics but also to millions worldwide. In 1858, before the emergence of the shrine, 14-year-old Bernadette Soubirous received visions of a beautiful lady, declared later to be the Virgin Mary. Lourdes receives more than five million pilgrims a year, many of them sick and disabled who bathe in its waters, hoping for recovery. Stories of medically authenticated cures such as the case of 32-year-old Marie

Bigot who suffered from blindness, deafness and hemiplegia, or 12-year-old Delizia Cirolli with bone tumour are only a part of the aura surrounding Lourdes. For over 120 years, the bureau's archives have recorded almost 7,000 supposed miraculous events. The Catholic Church has recognised approximately 70 as miracles.

At the time of writing, Dr Patrick Theillier, a GP of long-standing, is the doctor in charge of the Medical Bureau that studies alleged cures according to strict criteria. He maintains that a miracle must have a medical and spiritual dimension.[9] He describes the case of Jean-Pierre Bély who visited the shrine in 1987 when he was 36 after a long history of multiple sclerosis. Bély was confined to a wheelchair and on a full invalidity pension at the time. During the visit to Lourdes, he began to notice a return of sensation to his limbs and a few days later, he made a complete recovery. Theillier investigated Bély's case – a process that involved collecting statements from several medical experts who could confirm Bély's medical history. This material was then presented to the international medical committee of Lourdes, which consists of about 20 heads of European medical services. These people are believers, agnostics and atheists. The committee wanted to ensure that Bély was not suffering from a hysterical conversion type of disorder where an underlying psychological problem presents as a physical disorder without any physical pathology. Several psychiatrists testified that this was not the case.

According to Theillier, 99% of the people who come to Lourdes with their disease or handicap take it home with them, however 'they feel better here, almost inevitably, due to the climate of fraternity that exists here, the fact that they are being attended to, the love and tenderness that is lavished on them'.[10]

When I was a child, I stumbled on a book of Greek mythology. It was a fantastic discovery – fairy tales for adults. I loved the stories of the heroes and their superhuman qualities...Hercules, Achilles, and Perseus. Then of course, as I grew up, I realised there are other kinds of heroes. I realised that facing illness or any adversity demands qualities that are often greater than warrior skill. So my list of heroes grew, encompassing many everyday people. I call them my silent heroes. Stephanie is one of the many who brought her disease back home with her from Lourdes.

D: When did you first know that you were seriously ill?
Stephanie: I first knew that I was seriously ill when I was 14.
D: How did you manage to accept having the condition?
Stephanie: Well at the beginning, I didn't know that I had anything serious so I just put my strength into getting better. I thought it was going to be a temporary thing. My faith did come into it very early on because I realised that I wasn't going to be the same as everybody else. I remember when I first went for surgery. I couldn't sort of verbalise it at the time. It was only when I came

back that I remember feeling very strong and there is no reason why I should have done really but looking back I think I did feel some presence of God...sort of protected. I did have the strength of my family, obviously and they sort of enveloped me and looked after me but as things got worse there was a whole period of asking, 'Why God? Why me? Why do I have to go through this? I have learned so much from the experience but why do I have to carry on?' And then when I was probably at my lowest, I went to Lourdes and there I saw a completely different side to suffering. I saw people who had been ill all their lives who still managed to stay strong and I started to look at it in a completely different way. I wasn't thinking selfishly anymore and I started to see that I was part of a much bigger scheme of things really. Even that sort of sustained me for a short while because I had more companionship. I found a stronger faith but it kept me going for a short while but then I couldn't find it anywhere that wasn't Lourdes. I couldn't find it in the normal environment and people still felt very sorry for me even though I had this new-found faith.

[The following summer, Stephanie had a profound, life-changing spiritual experience that totally overwhelmed her. She felt 'sustained by spirituality'. It helped her relive the 'Lourdes experience' in everyday life.]

Stephanie: People even now say, 'How did you cope?' I'll say...the biggest thing I learned was that even though I felt very ill and useless, I could still give a contribution, I could still love. And even when I couldn't do anything at all, the way in which I was loved...the way in which I accepted it could be love for those people.

D: What do you mean when you say that spirituality enveloped you and what do you mean by love? Could you explain those two things to me?

Stephanie: The love thing...I think when I was first ill, if I had realised that I would always be ill, I would have thought my life would be useless and that I wouldn't achieve the things I had wanted to achieve. I wouldn't ever fulfil myself educationally. I would feel as if my life had stopped. Through meeting God, really, I realised that life isn't just about fulfilling ambitions and doing good things – it's how we make the most of what we have got. For me love is a Christian word and you can love everybody and anybody and it's a very positive thing. Even when life is very, very hard or even if somebody – it's difficult just saying it on the spot. For instance, if you're having a really awful test or something which is very, very unpleasant in my previous way of thinking it would just be something very, very unpleasant and I would just grit my teeth and get on it with it but thinking the new way, I could go through with that [the pain] for somebody or for something ... It wasn't something that would make me less but it was something that could make me better and could also be a gift to other people. It sounds very sentimental like that.

D: So it was more than just getting on with it. It was putting it into a different dimension.

Stephanie: Yes, and it wasn't important whether people knew that you were doing that. My benefit was that it made me strong and able to carry on but there was no selfish motive, if you know what I mean. There was no saying, 'well if I get on with this I'm going to be better' because I didn't know that or 'if I love this person, they are going to love me back' because they didn't necessarily know that. But it was something that made me feel that everything that I was doing was worthwhile even if nobody else knew that. It was that relationship with…well, God knew that. Nobody else knew that.

D: You said that when you went to Lourdes, you saw a different side to suffering. In what way did you see it?

Stephanie: My previous way of thinking before going to Lourdes was suffering is bad. There is nothing exceptionally good about suffering. It could perhaps teach you certain lessons, which I felt I had already learned, because it made me feel that a lot of things that I felt were important before I was ill, were no longer important. But in some ways it made me feel that health was even more important. I had just taken health for granted and then having gone through that experience I realised that you couldn't take health for granted but also a lot of attitudes had changed as well. You know, I felt that life just couldn't be the same again. When I went to Lourdes, it was different because I still felt that I was going to get better obviously but people there were crippled and maimed and blind and deaf and everything. Yes, I suppose I was seeing already this sort of aspect that they were still making their lives something good. They were still giving…they were still loving really but they probably didn't see it quite like that at the time.

D: You said as well that it seemed to fit into the experience of being part of a bigger whole. What do you mean by that?

Stephanie: I think it became obvious to me…that suffering is very much a part of life…life was never going to be without suffering. I didn't believe that anybody would not be touched by suffering. But it was what I did with the suffering that made me part of a bigger thing. And I think that very early on I realised this link with God. When he came to earth as a man, he suffered everything I had suffered and a lot more and I think that having that link with him, even if I felt abandoned by everyone else, I felt whole... I saw myself – not just because I had a physical illness but because everyone has some suffering – that my suffering had a name which was my illness but other people's suffering might not be named so easily…I think I understood that everyone has something…The way in which I lived my suffering could possibly help other people with the way that they lived theirs. They could perhaps see it not quite as useless a thing…am I explaining that?

D: What link would you see between spirituality and illness or between spirituality and health?

Stephanie: Well, for me, it's so linked.

D: What link would you see between the two? The way you are spiritually and the way you live your illness?

Stephanie: In that respect, I can see that when I am at my 'illest', when I have least, my spirituality always seems to be stronger, which is a constant thing and I try to constantly redress the balance. In a very strange way, when I thought that I was dying my spirituality could not have been stronger. I was so poor in health and so rich in spirituality. Most of the time, because there were times obviously when I was very, very low as well but it was like every emptiness had been filled and the more I lost, the more it was filled with God. In some ways, when I am more healthy, there isn't as much space for that spirituality and I have to constantly think, 'This isn't quite the way I want to live; I want to make more space for God'. So I actually have to cut things mentally rather…almost when I am illest – I have to abandon myself as well, it isn't something that just purely happens to me – I almost feel really sort of privileged. I suppose the more I empty myself, the more the emptiness is filled if I do it properly.

I had this conversation with a girl who has been exactly in the same position as me. She nearly died a couple of times and I said I was really quite frustrated because at that moment when I was prepared to die, my relationship with God was so strong I could touch him. I said, 'Why do I slip back when I am well?' And she said that she had had exactly the same experience. She said that she felt that in some way (it's so difficult to explain this properly) the nearer we are to death, the more we are prepared. We can't quite live like that all the time. It's almost not possible but we can just do our best. It's almost like a gift, that sort of light that you can have when you feel that you're at that point of almost death.

D: Would you say that the prayers of others have helped you?

Stephanie: Oh gosh! Absolutely…absolutely! It's happened all the way through at various points especially when I was in hospital but I think that the thing that demonstrates it most is that sort of final period when I was waiting for the transplant…it was the prayer that absolutely held me and it held everybody around me as well. At those moments where I would perhaps have given up totally – and if I had have given up, there is no doubt I would have died – I had to go along with the treatment.

D: What was the chance of you getting a transplant?

Stephanie: Nobody could actually quite answer that question. There were so few transplants being done at that time. For some reason there was an incredible lack of donors and what made it even more apparent to me that I wouldn't get one was that when I went into hospital those few months before I got my transplant about nine patients died in one two week period…nine patients died!

D: All awaiting transplant…

Stephanie: All of them awaiting transplant. And there were a few who because they realised that it was hopeless, they just took their oxygen masks off and…

D: They just gave up…

Stephanie: It sounds as if they just gave up but they were so…

D: They were too ill…

Stephanie: They were so ill. They required so much energy and effort to try...the fact that they could just leave their oxygen mask off and just slip away – obviously they were so near to death. And I think for me, it was only the one time that I felt it was so physically tiring…I mean you had no energy anyway and it took you so much energy to even eat. It would take you an hour to eat what would take a normal person five minutes and that sheer amount of effort to do every little bit of treatment which was the only thing that was keeping you alive.

D: But what helped you go on? Something must have driven you to go on…to continue. What do you think of that?

Stephanie: Well, I was going to say there was one particular day when I decided…I knew in my own mind that I preferred to die. I had done all those steps that I wanted to do – all the most important steps. I had said 'goodbye' to people, told people that I loved them, said my prayers, had the 'blessing of the sick' [special rite administered by a priest to someone who is seriously ill] – all these steps… And on this particular day when physio came to treat me (which was a very important part of the treatment obviously) she asked if she could treat me and I said 'no' and she didn't persuade me. She didn't even try and she spent that time with me and went away and I suddenly thought to myself – I was sitting there quietly – I still thought I was going to die, I almost had no doubt in my own mind. For me I thought the end was going to be inevitable anyway, but I was very, very aware of all this prayer that was going on around me and I thought, if I was going to die I wanted it to be because there was no other way. I didn't want to die because I had given up and from somewhere – I think probably from the prayer all around me – I managed to grab that last bit of strength and start again. And the strange thing was that the very next day was the day that I got the call for the transplant. It was as if God knew that I had used my very last reserve and that this was my last chance really.

The one thing that helped me through the whole of the illness was this idea of the 'present moment'. I think that sometimes when I couldn't think a long time ahead – you know, maybe I had a pneumonia or a very bad infection or whatever or I could hardly breathe, let alone think – I couldn't have thought about next week or tomorrow but I could think of that present moment and it was lots of 'present moments' strung together that got me through so many, many times.

What I have never understood – and there were several people who I met when I was in hospital who would say that they didn't believe and the things that they overcame, the times that they nearly died…there were a few times – especially when I was in intensive care after the transplant – when I couldn't pray. I did feel totally lost in the wilderness, but it was those times when…I was just totally blocked…and my friend came and she said, 'I'll say your prayers for you'. It was then when I was totally lost that I did rely on other people to take over…

It has been like an apprenticeship

Cervical cancer is the sixth most common malignancy in females and every year there are 16 new cases in 100,000 women. It mainly occurs in women aged 45 to 55. The prognosis is better in more industrialised countries because cervical screening catches the condition at a very early stage.

Forty-three-year-old Diana is a philosophy teacher and this is her story.

> I can divide my life into two parts. The first part lasted 38 years and during that time, I grew up, went to university in the big city and stayed on after I graduated. During that long period, I faced all sorts of crises. I have had problems with religion since I was a young girl and did not know what to do with my life. We all face these problems but some get through them more easily than others do. I am one of those people who occasionally come to a dead end. Besides, it was difficult for me to find the perfect partner. I was full of ideals but you come up against reality in life and not idealism. Growing up was hard for me. It was hard to find happiness and peace. It was hard for me not to be too self-critical…
>
> Well, perhaps you'll ask where this is all leading. It is quite simple really. Five years ago, a miracle began to happen. Something totally unexpected happened and it turned everything upside down. My ordered, rather dutiful, lonely, unhappy life, played out in my head, was upset by a cancer diagnosis. Now I can speak of the five years 'post cancer'. It has been like an apprenticeship where I have learned about courage and love. I have learned how to let myself be loved and how to love. I have learned that this love includes not only people who are close by and family but also friends, friends of friends, acquaintances and strangers, human beings and other forms of life including nature and the entire Universe. So I have found God through love and love is a sacred force.
>
> …Love is the powerful force that protects us from everything we fear and it makes us discover inside courage we never dreamed we had. Love is one of God's many names.

The pain of being human

Perhaps the famous cellist Jacqueline Du Pré is one of the musicians most associated with a medical condition. The music that she made was thrilling – she said that playing 'lifts you out of yourself into a delirious place'.[11] Du Pré epitomised all that is talented and promising. She was wantonly struck down at the height of her career by a devastating illness – multiple sclerosis (MS). It is the most common cause of neurological disability in young adults. It is a condition of loss: loss of mobility in the limbs, loss of sensation in the fingers and feet, loss of balance, loss of bladder control...

In the poem 'ms' David Watts tries to help us feel some of the neuropathy symptoms of a sufferer:

> ...it felt like oatmeal
> drying on the skin
> only with oats you can see
> where the damage is...
> ...while this moth of his nightmare
> kept eating at the wool
> of his nerve endings[12]

Tina is an elderly woman who suffers from a condition with effects similar to MS. Her symptoms appeared dramatically.

I feel very diffident talking about myself and illness. I think really the word is suffering – illness is 'suffering'. Suffering is universal – we all – you all – have suffered or are suffering. And it's very personal. It's hard to describe, to pinpoint where the suffering is greatest – the physical: where and how? (You know how people sometimes say 'on a scale of 1-10 where do you come? Well one is no pain and ten presumably endless pain – so you make a dive at a number. Five is fairly safe.) Or mental suffering – and that sounds fairly daft, but it's very real.

I do have an illness and it's called neuropathy (which means dying nerves and therefore muscles). I walk with difficulty as my feet, legs and low back have no muscles to help. It's a bit like MS or muscular dystrophy. I have had it for 25 years and it is progressive.

I used to be quite strong physically and whatever I asked my body to do – it did it! I was a doer rather than a thinker or a 'be-er'. The disability struck me very rapidly. One day I was busy 'doing' and the next morning as I got out of bed – nothing worked! My feet were all over the place and I had no strength. I was shocked (and scared) but recovered quickly because I never contemplated for a single second that it was something that couldn't be put right by doctors. It just didn't enter my head that it could be anything that couldn't be fixed. I was young(ish) and had a lot to learn!

I was a Christian and here, suddenly I had to face up to something else. So my journey began and from time to time – out of frustration and pain I would weep and forget that my heart needed enlarging and that God did love me immensely. I was filled with a very human emotion of fear and a longing to be able to control my own life. But in the very act of weeping and breaking and being pitched into darkness – darkness from which there appeared to be no escape – I knew somewhere inside myself that there was a way out if I could only let go…and allow God to take me over. I seem to be speaking about the pain of being human – and how I seek to live out that pain.

Spiritual experiences are not just induced by chronic illness and suffering, but also by acute ones. The experience of Alexei Alexandrovich Karenin, the husband of Anna Karenin, is such an example. The story is set in nineteenth century Russia and the characters are from the upper echelons of society. Alexei Alexandrovich Karenin is in an impossible situation. His wife has been unfaithful to him and is pregnant with her lover's child. After childbirth, she develops puerperal fever and the prognosis is abysmal with 99% mortality. Karenin goes to see his wife, having decided that he will divorce her – hopeful even that she will die and therefore avoid the shame and scandal of divorce. Karenin, a cold man, fears display of raw emotion – particularly tears. Anna is delirious and in her ravings, babbles about her remorse and begs forgiveness of Karenin who is overwhelmed by a deep spiritual experience:

> He suddenly felt that what he had regarded as nervous agitation was on the contrary a blissful spiritual condition that gave him all at once a new happiness he had never known…a glad feeling of love and forgiveness for his enemies filled his heart…By his sick wife's bedside he had given way for the first time in his life to that feeling of sympathetic compassion which the suffering of others produced in him, and which he had hitherto been ashamed of, as of a pernicious weakness…He suddenly felt that the very thing that was the source of his sufferings had become the source of his spiritual joy.[13]

One of the oldest stories about illness is the Book of Job in the Bible. The Book of Job is one of the Wisdom Books, the fruit of a movement among ancient oriental people to garner and express the results of human experience in order to understand and solve life's problems. In the story – which to some extent could be the story of every person who suffers – the writer tries to address the fundamental, existential, six billion dollar question. Why is there suffering and – if there has to be suffering – why do the innocent, why do good people suffer?

Today we are not so different. We ask the same questions about life, suffering and death. Questions like those posed by Job, a prosperous, righteous, God-fearing man. God delights in the goodness of his 'servant Job'. Satan (which means 'adversary') however, points out that Job can afford to be God-fearing because he is wealthy. Satan is convinced that if Job suffers, he is bound to turn against God.

Job then suffers a terrible reversal of fortune and loses his children and property. A horrible disease afflicts his body. He despairs:

Vermin and loathsome scabs cover my body; my skin is cracked and oozes
pus.
Swifter than a weaver's shuttle my days have passed, and vanished, leaving
no hope behind.

Job, 7:5 and 6[14]

He is not a docile, resigned sufferer but he questions the meaning of his existence and wishes that he had never been born:

Perish the day on which I was born and the night that told of a boy
conceived…
Why was I not still-born, or why did I not perish as I left the womb?
Why give light to a man of grief? Why give life to those bitter of heart,
Who long for a death that never comes, and hunt for it more than for buried
treasure.

Job 3:3, 11, 20, and 21[14]

Job's friends try to rationalise his suffering, ascribing the cause to some latent
sin. They say that his suffering must be deserved as they equate good fortune
with a blameless life. Job refuses to accept this idea and continues to question.
God eventually answers Job and although God does not give a reason for his
suffering, Job recognises that he has dealt with things he does not understand…too wonderful for him to know. He concludes, 'I had heard of you by
word of mouth, but now my eyes have seen you.' Job emerges from his experience a wealthier man than he was before and not just materially. It is as if suffering has served as a catalyst for his spiritual growth and development to a
greater extent than that allowed by the prosperity and good fortune of his life
before.

SPIRITUAL METAMORPHOSIS

At the beginning of this chapter, we explored Gregor Samsa's metamorphosis.
Job too has a metamorphosis but it is not only physical. It involves his whole
being and he questions the meaning of his existence. Gregor never seems to ask
deeply the meaning of his suffering – perhaps he cannot articulate the question. Job rages against his pain. Gregor shuts his eyes in death while Job
manages to acquire new eyes.

From the patient narratives, it is obvious that for each one there was a metamorphosis akin to Gregor's and Job's. The themes present in the stories were
consistent with Renetzky's definition of the spiritual dimension referred to in
Chapter 2:

The 'power within man' giving 'meaning, purpose and fulfilment' to life, suffering and death; the individual's 'will to live'; the individual's belief and faith in self, others and God.[15]

Meaning

Illness tended to precipitate all of those interviewed into a state where they had to examine the meaning of their illness and of their very existence. Some had asked themselves those questions before but only superficially. Finding a meaning led to acceptance, endurance, hope and in some cases compliance with medication and therefore better 'health' physically, emotionally, psychologically and socially. Anna for example says that God is very important to her and gives meaning to everything she does and not just to her illness:

> Well, everything I do, I try to do what is best...He is just important. Like...if I do something, like trying to do it right for God.

Helen's complete narrative is not featured in this book but she too struggles to make sense of her illness. She has virtual paralysis of all her limbs because of MS and at 35 needs help with basic things such as toileting and dressing. She comments wryly that she could not even shift the annoying strand of hair that brushed against her lashes as she blinked. She is attractive, vivacious and full of good humour. Her spiritual life is the only thing that gives her any sense of meaning, although it is not always easy: 'for this absurd situation, there has to be some reason.'

Sense of purpose in life

The narratives also reveal the need for a sense of purpose in life with underlying themes such as:
➤ the feeling of a driving force within
➤ seeing the relationship of illness to spiritual life
➤ an ascetic view of life and death
➤ 'sort of philosophy' necessary to go on.

Linda stipulates that she does not believe in the existence of any divine power or force, yet she is equally insistent that 'Somebody decides what purpose we live for'. This sense of purpose gives her the will to live, has positive effects on her health and helps her overcome moments of crisis in her illness.

Some saw illness as a punishment or a way of atoning for the sins of others. Molly comments, 'Now, they always say, don't they, that if you're suffering on earth, you're paying for somebody's sins.' While Margaret racks her brains, trying to understand what she has done wrong with her life to deserve cancer. They are both religious people, but Linda who is not a churchgoer, also echoes her partner's words, 'Bill used to say "Why you? Of all people, you've never done anything."'

Will to live

Each person interviewed has a strong will to live. Common themes are:
➤ being a fighter
➤ courage
➤ determination
➤ extraordinary strength.

Lucy survived against the odds and amazed the medical profession. One of the doctors caring for her commented that she was the strongest child that he had ever met.

Belief and faith in self, others, God

Linda does not have any religious affiliation but she does have a strong belief and faith in herself. This gives her the determination to go on. This faith in herself and the relationship with her family keeps her alive. Instead, despite her diagnosis, Lucy has an unshakeable belief in God and prayer.

Renetzky's definition of the spiritual dimension seems to be apparent in the narratives. However, it is only part of the story. Spirituality is not just an entity isolated to what the we experience within, but it is also manifest in how we live the experience of life, illness and suffering – the 'consequential dimension' as Ndlela says.[3] This dimension of spirituality is apparent in additional themes that surfaced from the narratives:
➤ refocussing, prioritising and changing of perspective
➤ more understanding and tolerance
➤ being a greater listener
➤ 'here and now'
➤ altruism.

Confined to a wheelchair, Helen shares how her experience of illness has led to a change in perspective:

> It is realising the priorities of life are not just putting on mascara. Things have to become simpler.

Seventy-year-old Thomas had treatment in hospital several years ago for prostate cancer. His illness helped him refocus on his spiritual life:

> To be quite honest, you notice things more in a period in hospital...in a period of enforced rest there is almost an opportunity for spirituality to – it's not that you

don't live it but you are so busy doing what you have to do in your ordinary life that you forget...

Greater understanding and tolerance, as well as the capacity to listen more to others are other themes that emerge from the interviews as elements of spirituality. Margaret feels that through suffering from throat cancer, she has learned to listen more to others while Lucy feels that she understands others better, 'no matter what people have got or their appearance changed, don't criticise them'.

Importance of the here and now

Helen, Stephanie, Anna and all the others show me that spirituality is not simply an emotion, idea, sentiment or philosophy but also a way of life. How they lived with their illness to some extent mirrored their spiritual dimension. Linda for example says that she values time more because she does not know how much she has and it is 'really precious', while Helen, speaks about living the 'present moment':

> ...for years I have always thought it sensible to live the present...I have had a decade of illness. If I had known things would have been so difficult I would have been having none of it.

Stephanie states that focussing on the present helped her through the whole of her illness, particularly when she was very ill following transplant surgery. She tried not to think of the past or future but to 'concentrate on living fully now'.

The importance of the here and now is not a new concept. In a Latin poem, Horace exhorts us to 'seize the day' (carpe diem) while Buddha suggests, 'Do not dwell in the past, do not dream of the future, concentrate the mind on the present moment.' He also says

> The secret of health for both mind and body is not to mourn for the past, nor to worry about the future, but to live the present moment wisely and earnestly.[16]

Abraham Maslow believes the ability to be in the present moment is a major component of mental wellness. While Blaise Pascal, the seventeenth century philosopher, has much to say about the value of being focussed on the present, confirming what our storytellers learnt from their illness experience:

> We never keep to the present. We recall the past; we anticipate the future as if we found it too slow in coming and we were trying to hurry it up, or we recall the past as if to stay its too rapid flight. We are so unwise that we wander about in times that do not belong to us, and do not think of the only one that does; so vain that

we dream of times that are not and blindly flee the only one that is. The fact is that the present usually hurts. We thrust it out of sight because it distresses us, and if we find it enjoyable, we are sorry to see it slip away. We try to give it the support of the future, and think how we are going to arrange things over which we have no control, for a time we can never be sure of reaching.[17]

Illness focusses sufferers on the unavoidable present. There is enforced inactivity and endless hours spent propped up against a hospital waiting room wall. There is the suspense of long-awaited test results that never seem to be available at a follow-up appointment...

Those who suffer are compelled to face the pain of the present moment and therefore they can truly live....

Let each of us examine his thoughts; he will find them wholly concerned with the past or the future. We almost never think of the present; and if we think of it, it is only to see what light it throws on our plans for the future. The present is never our end. The past and the present are our means, the future alone our end. Thus we never actually live, but hope to live, and since we are always planning how to be happy, it is inevitable we should never be so.[17]

Living fully immersed in the present means different things to different people. From the narratives it is not a carefree *'che sarà, sarà'* attitude but it means taking on the pain of the present – something deeply spiritual.

Beyond philanthropy

In Maslow's hierarchy of needs, self-actualisation occupies the tip of the pyramid while our essential physiological needs form the base. Safety, love, belonging and esteem lie in between.

Maslow considered that in almost every human being there is an active will toward health, a drive towards growth, or towards the fulfilment of human potentialities.[18] For Maslow, self-actualizing people live more independently of their basic needs and they are more ego transcending. They reach such a high level of maturation, health and self-fulfilment that they almost seem like a breed apart. Self-actualising people deeply identify with others, feeling intense empathy, compassion and affection for other people and for human beings generally. Self-actualising people have experiences of transcendence that may be intensely spiritual.

With the Dalai Lama, compassion and love are not 'peak' experiences, but are the essentials for our very existence:

Love and compassion are necessities, not luxuries. Without them humanity cannot survive.

The narratives disclose how focussing on others was helpful in coping with illness. The illness experience heightened the sensitivity to others and the ability to empathise with them. It gave some of the sufferers a greater sense of benevolence, kindness and feeling of humanity towards others. In this way, it enhanced their spirituality.

Helen says that her illness sometimes gives her the 'feeling of being an exile' from her real self. It is physically impossible for her to cuddle her young nieces and nephews, but then she finds great solace in loving them 'with all my limits'. For her, this consists of 'tuning into people; understanding where they're coming from; not being overbearing about my situation; trying to lighten life.'

Thomas remarks that focussing on other people and their needs during his stay in hospital were of such fundamental importance to him because it helped him step outside himself and forget himself and his situation:

> ...it helped me to communicate with a man with a tracheostomy who couldn't talk, put up with the TV blaring, and respect the silence of another who wouldn't talk.

Stephanie remarks that channelling her thoughts on the sufferings of other people helps her manage the difficult moments of her own illness.

Tina and Stephanie describe their spiritual experience in terms of a journey. Margaret and Molly tend to emphasise the intellectual and ritualistic dimension of spirituality more. However, between them, they all have elements of both models that Kliewer and Saultz present for studying spirituality (intellectual, ideological, ritualistic, experiential, consequential and supportive aspects and the quest).[3] From the stories it is evident that each patient sets off on a quest – unwittingly or intentionally – and comes back altered. Unlike Gregor Samsa, they are not stuck in the chrysalis bug stage of the journey but they emerge transformed, spiritually enriched by the illness experience.

Veronica Towers wrote this song for a friend who was dying of cancer. Veronica had searched everywhere for cherries – her friend's favourite fruit – but it was impossible to obtain them because it was too early in the year. So she wrote this song, which encapsulates her story and the other stories and experiences, which I have been privileged to hear:

> It's not the time of year for cherries
> now is the time for other fruit
> and all your flowers fall like blossom
> while we can only watch with you.
>
> Yet in your eyes I've seen a vision
> no longer glimpses of the truth,

of all that's real and all that matters,
where wisdom shines as bright as youth.

And is pain the way we wash the
windows of our eyes?
Why is losing the only way to find?[19]

Perhaps I was too hard on Gregor Samsa when I said at the beginning of the chapter that he did not really ask himself the meaning of his existence and of his suffering. Perhaps he could not articulate these questions because he remained an alien in the eyes of his family and of other people. He was devoid of the acceptance and warmth that he needed to move beyond the 'chrysalis' stage. Stephanie, Anna, Lucy, Tina and all the others made strides in their spiritual journeys encouraged by the support of family, friends, carers and – in some cases – healthcare professionals.

Professional carers and medical staff alleviate physical pain, treat illness, offer support with mental health problems and look to the local minister or hospital chaplain to give spiritual assistance. Chaplains are, after all, experts in this area. However, what if doctors and nurses attribute suffering in a patient to physical pathology when in fact the problem is a spiritual one? What if the patient's depression is at an impasse not because of the 'wrong medication' but because of an unidentified and unrecognised spiritual crisis? What if the patient does not feel motivated to take medication because life has no meaning? With such possible scenarios, healthcare professionals are obliged at least to recognise the spiritual dimension in their patients so they offer appropriate support and therapy. Spiritual distress and tools that may help its recognition is the topic of the next chapter.

REFERENCES

1 Narrative based medicine. Tavistock Clinic. www.tavi-port.org
2 Kafka F. *Metamorphosis*. London: Penguin Books; 2006.
3 Kliewer SP, Saultz J. *Healthcare and Spirituality*. Oxford: Radcliffe Publishing; 2005.
4 Gilliam Fisher D. 'Sixty-five Roses'. *One of Everything*. Cleveland: Cleveland State University Poetry Center; 2003.
5 Gilliam Fisher D. 'Crescendo, Descrescendo'. *One of Everything*. Cleveland: Cleveland State University Poetry Center; 2003.
6 Kovner A. *Sloan Kettering*. Berlin: Schocken; 2002.
7 Milton J. *Encyclopaedia Britannica*. London: Encyclopaedia Britannica; 2008.
8 Beethoven L. *Beethoven's Letters 1790–1826, Volume 1*. Wallace Lady G, translator. 1866.
9 Theillier P. *Talking About Miracles*. Alton: Redemptorist Publications; 2004.
10 Spinney L. 'Miracle worker'. The *Guardian*. 30 September 2004.
11 Du Pré J. www.brainyquote.com/quotes/authors/j/jacqueline_du_pre.html

12 Watts D. *Taking the History*. Troy: Nightshade Press; 1999.

13 Tolstoy L. *Anna Karenina*. Edmonds R, translator. London: Penguin Classics; 1975.

14 Book of Job. *New Jerusalem Bible*. London: Darton, Longman & Todd; 1985.

15 Renetzky L. The fourth dimension: applications to the social services. In: Moberg D, editor. *Spiritual Well-being: sociological perspectives*. Washington: University Press of America; 1979.

16 www.brainyquote.com/quotes/quotes/b/buddha121785.html

17 Pascal B. *Pensées*. Krailsheimer AJ, translator. London: Penguin Classics; 1966.

18 Maslow A. *The Farther Reaches of Human Nature*. London: Penguin Books; 1973.

19 Towers V. *Promises of Life*. CD produced by Simon Heyworth; 2002.

Spiritual distress

'Man – a being in search of meaning.'
Plato

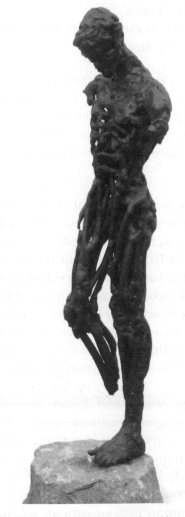

Daniel (an AIDs sufferer) by Lau Hung

SPIRITUAL DIMENSION AND THE HEALTHCARE PROFESSIONAL

As I tore off the wrapping of a magazine recently, a few fliers fell to the ground. The words of a patient written on one of them immediately captured my attention: 'A good doctor removes 50% of the illness just by talking.'[1] I believe this although I am not sure in every instance that doctors help remove 50%. It is true that doctors, healthcare professionals and carers potentially do much to relieve suffering just by the way they are. Conversely, they may do much to increase suffering. However, 'talking' is not simply giving a nice detailed explanation nor supplying people with reams of literature about their condition. I think the 'talking' to which this patient is referring is communication that empathises with the patient. You talk to the other, as you would like to be treated if you were in his place. You talk to the patient as if you identified with his pain. A Cheyenne proverb advises us not to judge another until we have walked 'two moons in his moccasins.'

Illness causes suffering. Illness causes devastation. Virginia Woolf describes the spiritual change wrought by illness:

> Considering how common illness is, how tremendous the spiritual change that it brings, how astonishing, when the lights of health go down...what wastes and deserts of the soul a slight attack of influenza brings to view...when we think of this, as we are so frequently forced to think of it, it becomes strange indeed that illness has not taken its place with love and battle and jealousy among the prime themes of literature.[2]

Studies have demonstrated that most people have a spiritual life and most patients want their spiritual needs assessed and addressed. This may be so, but is it important? It appears to be. Researchers found the subscale, which looks at existential well-being in the McGill quality of life questionnaire, is an important predictor of the quality of life. Studies have also shown a link between the spiritual dimension and health outcomes. An example is a study of thirty Islamic patients who had suffered bereavement. Fifteen were assigned to a control group where they were given psychotherapy and fifteen received psychotherapy with support – which included readings from the Koran – for their religious beliefs. At the end of six months, the second group had shown greater and faster improvement.[3]

After controlling for age, gender and disease severity, a further group of researchers also found that religious involvement was likely to play an important role in altering the pain experience of patients with Sickle-Cell Disease. Attending church once or more times each week was associated with lower measures of pain. They concluded that religion might be an important area for the future study of other populations of chronically ill patients.[4]

In the USA, apparently up to 77% of patients would like spiritual issues considered as part of their package of care while only 10% to 20% of doctors actually discuss them.[5] A paper from the Mayo Clinic gives the following reasons for acknowledging and supporting the spiritual dimension in patients.

➤ Patients regard their spiritual and physical health of equal importance.
➤ Research suggests that good spiritual health improves coping and quality of life during illness. It may also be a source of identity, meaning, purpose, hope, reassurance and transcendence and thus lessen the uncertainties of illness.
➤ Acknowledging and addressing the spiritual dimension may enhance cultural sensitivity.
➤ Supporting the patient's spiritual health may improve the doctor-patient relationship.
➤ As the doctor's task is to cure disease where possible and to relieve suffering always, addressing spiritual health should be regarded in the same light as tackling psychosocial factors that affect the delivery of care and the outcomes of illness.[6]

It therefore follows that supporting spiritual health may improve coping and recovery from illness. Besides patients may feel that medicine has nothing to offer them if their spiritual dimension is not addressed. Research in California looked at the medical records of 172 children who died over a twenty-year period because their parents withdrew medical care and relied on religious rituals. Sadly, 140 of the children died of conditions where the expected survival with routine medical care was estimated at over 90%.[7] Perhaps if the medical and nursing staff had recognised the importance of incorporating the spiritual dimension in the care of the children and their families, some of these deaths would have been avoided.

Nonetheless, not all of us are comfortable talking about spiritual matters. In her witty book, *Watching the English*, Kate Fox states the English display a benign indifference to God's existence and that this indifference remains unaltered as long as they are not embarrassed or bored by the religious zeal of a minority. She says that any mention of God is 'improper display' while 'earnestness of any kind makes us squirm...makes us deeply suspicious and decidedly twitchy'.[8]

Uneasiness talking about religion and spirituality is of course not just found in some English people. Many other people the world over feel uncomfortable. *Many healthcare workers feel uncomfortable.* Western fiction in the nineteenth and twentieth century at times depicts doctors as indifferent or hostile towards religion. Dr Denis Minoret in Balzac's *Ursule Minoret* and Dr Fortunati (alias Beelzebub) in *The Nun's Story* by Kathryn Hulme are such examples. In AJ Cronin's the *Keys of the Kingdom* there is the good doctor Mitchell who is a determined atheist much to the chagrin of his friend Fr Chisolm. Literature portrays the doctor as the rationalist with the sound scientific mind. Consequently, the good citizens of George Eliot's Middlemarch have no confidence in religious doctors:[9]

> The Doctor [Dr Sprague] was more than suspected of having no religion, but somehow Middlemarch tolerated this deficiency in him as if he had been a Lord Chancellor; indeed it is probable that his professional weight was the more believed in...At all events, it is certain that if any medical man had come to Middlemarch with the reputation of having very definite religious views, of being given to prayer, and of otherwise showing an active piety, there would have been a general presumption against his medical skill.

Medicine has progressed enormously since George Eliot's time. There have been colossal technological strides over the last fifty years. We have the MRI scanner, laser surgery, organ transplantation and an array of tools and tomes of knowledge at our disposal. Despite the tools designed to bring the doctor closer to the patient's problems, the doctor risks becoming ever more distant. One of the chief limitations of technological medicine is that in the relentless search for cures for disease, human suffering is somewhat neglected. The risk follows that if suffering is seen as serving no real purpose, it is either ignored or banished.[10]

THE WOUNDED HEALER

Chiron (or Cheiron) in the stories of Greek mythology is a centaur who is a healer and hunter. He instructed many of the heroes of ancient Greece. He taught them hunting but he also taught Asclepius – often depicted with a serpent-entwined staff – medicine. Chiron himself was wounded accidentally with one of Hercules' poisoned arrows. The wounded healer could not heal himself. He too is vulnerable.

So what happens if a doctor becomes unwell? What happens when suffering makes all the deeper questions about life's meaning emerge? Robert Klitzman looked at precisely this. He undertook in-depth interviews with 70 doctors who became sick. He discovered that doctors found it difficult to take on the role of patients and, at times, there was denial – some feeling marginalised by their colleagues. Sadly, some even experienced discrimination. He also found that sick doctors came to appreciate the value of the spiritual dimension. The doctors seemed to fall into groups who:

➤ were spiritual to start with
➤ experienced 'spirituality' despite themselves
➤ were spiritual, but not thinking of themselves as such
➤ wanted but were unable to believe
➤ continued to doubt
➤ played the game: ritual without acknowledging belief.[11]

Klitzman describes how an HIV sufferer had a strong desire to be more spiritual and felt the need of a firmer faith to help him cope with his illness despite his scepticism:

I just have this darn sceptical...on the one hand, I want and need it; on the other, I feel it's what weak, simple people rely on: a crutch.

Another doctor felt that scientific training promoted this scepticism as he found it hard to reconcile the rational world of science and the irrational world of religion and spirituality:

I'm looking for a spiritual component, but I tend to be kind of agnostic. I wish I weren't...but I have such a scientific bent, and organised religion, and most people out there who believe that, with their crystals...it's such a turnoff. It's difficult for me to open up to it. I'm trying to be open to that...It just seems like it's just a more successful way to live.

THE PATIENT'S PERSPECTIVE

Someone once came to see me alarmed about pain in his knee. He was healthy and in his early thirties. He had done a long hike up and down a mountain with some friends and had just about managed to keep up with their hectic pace. The next day he had persistent knee pain. There had been no bony injury and there was no swelling in the joint, which seemed sturdy. While I examined him, various diagnostic possibilities flitted into my head and out again as I summarily discarded them.

I smiled at him – I thought reassuringly – satisfied there was nothing seriously wrong with the knee. There was no answering smile. He was not satisfied with my explanations about a muscle or ligament sprain. In fact, when I looked at him more closely, I could see that he was quite anxious. I realised that I had worked out a meaning for his knee pain with which I was content. He was not! As I probed further, I understood what the knee pain meant to him. For the first time in his life, he had not only experienced morbidity, imagining 'degeneration' and 'incapacity' but he had also glimpsed his mortality. I realised that this had 'freaked him out'. I recognized too that no explanation that I could give him about the benign nature of the knee problem would reassure him unless I in some way addressed his underlying existential fear.

Kliewer and Saultz[12] recommend a multifaceted approach on assessing patients – multifaceted and complex beings who need to be treated holistically. They give the example of a woman consulting a doctor with severe arthritis in her hands. She is unable to continue her work as a musician and is limited in many other activities. The doctor will focus on her hands but it is critical that 'the healer also understand what is happening in the other facets of the patient's personhood'. On a physical level there is arthritis, emotionally the patient feels a sense of worthlessness and valuelessness, socially there is isolation, while spiritually she feels disconnected from God. Each facet may be having an impact on the others and so simply scoring the pain level on a scale from one to ten will only give a partial idea of the patient's health: 'to treat patients from only the biomedical perspective is to turn them into a cadaver'.[12]

It seems obvious to state but it may be quickly forgotten that a patient is a person. Vera Araujo defines a person as a rational individual who has a relationship with three elements: the Absolute, fellow humans and the cosmos. For her the word 'individual' is too poor a description of the person as it is an abstract almost self-contained unit. Instead, the term 'person' is loaded with identity, charged with values and replete with culture, history and relationships.[13] Patients are not objects or interesting cases of kidney or heart disease. As patients are people and as healthcare workers are people, we relate to one another through relationships. This is rudimentary, but the stories that people tell of visits to hospitals and doctor's surgeries, at times show that they have not been treated as people.

What patients want from healthcare workers

Illness comes with many questions. We ask, 'Why me?' 'What will happen?' 'Will I die?' 'What does it mean?' We are also afraid of the dark:

> Illness is the night-side of life, a more onerous citizenship. Everyone who is born holds dual citizenship. In the kingdom of the well and in the kingdom of the sick. Although we all prefer to use only the good passport, sooner or later each of us is obliged, at least for a spell, to identify as citizens of that other place.[14]

In a focus study group, 22 patients hospitalised for life-threatening illnesses considered excellent bedside manner, empathy and communication skills to be necessary for spiritual assessment. Some wished for this assessment to take place within the context of routine medical care and others considered that it should evolve from the stress of being ill. Some did not wish to have any spiritual assessment for fear the doctor would impose his own beliefs or that such an assessment was a herald for disaster in the form of a poor prognosis.[15,16]

Another study by Narayanasamy explored the spiritual 'mechanisms' that patients adopt to help them cope with chronic illness. The author found the following coping mechanisms:

➤ reaching out to God in the belief and faith that help will be forthcoming (plea for help)
➤ feeling connected to God through prayer (having a dialogue with God, remonstration)
➤ searching for meaning and purpose (questions about life and impact of illness, existence)
➤ strategy of privacy (sense of loneliness, fear of being ridiculed)
➤ connectedness with others (family, spiritual resources).

The study concluded that patients might benefit from nursing interventions that are sensitive, supportive and responsive to their spiritual needs.[17]

In the Midlands, UK, 22 hospital patients recorded accounts of their experience of spiritual distress. They also spoke about their hopes for spiritual wholeness. The patients were receiving palliative or other forms of therapy and the responses in the two groups were virtually the same. Spiritual distress focussed most frequently around the sense of not being themselves, of 'dis-integrity'. Instead, the hope to help others and using the illness as a vehicle for personal growth and acceptance were seen as paths to spiritual wholeness (integrity). Interestingly, the patients considered support from hospital staff as crucial to facilitating the change from distress to integrity.[18]

Spiritual wholeness

There are many examples in literature of how spiritual wholeness results in better health. Pollyanna Whittier is an illustration. She is an 11-year old orphan thrust on to the care of her stuffy aunt. Her bright optimistic nature warms hearts, spreads sunshine and harmony. One of her many protégées is Mrs Snow who sounds something of a hypochondriac as she alternately lies listlessly on her pillow and sits upright when Pollyanna surprises her with some sharp, innocent observation about her. Pollyanna's answer to any adversity, to all the vicissitudes of life, is to be glad that things are not worse than they are – the *glad game*. Mrs Snow snappishly challenges Pollyanna to think about something that she can be glad about as she is confined to her bed all day. Pollyanna *does* think: Mrs Snow can be glad that other people do not have to be sick all day in bed like her.

Pollyanna is involved in a road accident. She lies immobile in bed. True to her nature, she is glad that she does not have smallpox (as this is worse than freckles), glad that she does not have whooping cough, appendicitis or measles. She then hears accidentally that she will never be able to walk and wonders how she will ever be glad about anything again. She becomes utterly miserable and depressed. The whole town learns to play the game and is 'wonderfully happier'. Pollyanna comes to learn this. She then decides there *is* something she can be glad about after all, 'I can be glad I've had my legs, anyway – else I couldn't have done – that!'[19]

Another children's book, *The Secret Garden*,[20] is on the surface a tale about three youngsters who give life to an abandoned desolate garden. Two of the children – Mary and Colin – are damaged and sick. The transformation of the garden parallels the change that takes place in both of them. For example, when Mary's mind

> filled itself with robins, and moorland cottages crowded with children…with springtime and with secret gardens coming alive day by day…there was no room left for the disagreeable thoughts which affected her liver and her digestion and made her yellow and tired.

Similarly, as long as Colin shut himself up in his room absorbed in his fears, weakness and limitations, reflecting

> hourly on humps and early death, he was a hysterical, half-crazy little hypo-chondriac who knew nothing of the sunshine and the spring and also did not know that he could get well and could stand upon his feet if he tried to do it.

The real 'doctor' of the story is Dickon – the boy gardener who befriends Mary and Colin – not the family doctor. Dickon is the wise healer. Mary and later Colin recognise that Dickon worked 'good Magic' on the garden and on people around him. The children are transformed physically, emotionally and spiritually. Colin astutely says one day

> There must be lots of Magic in the world, but people don't know what it is like or how to make it. Perhaps the beginning is just to say nice things are going to happen until you make them happen. I am going to try and experiment.

THE DOCTOR'S PERSPECTIVE
The art of medicine
Sir Arthur Conan Doyle is best known for his literary creations Sherlock Holmes and Dr Watson. He was also a general practitioner and in a collection of short stories, he describes some scenes reminiscent of medicine today. Dr Winter in 'Behind the Times' is one of the characters whom he seems secretly to admire. Winter scorns the stethoscope and would still bleed patients if he could. Despite this, his patients do very well:

> He has the healing touch – that magnetic thing which defies explanation or analysis, but which is a very evident fact none the less. His mere presence leaves the patient with more hopefulness and vitality...He would shoo Death out of the room as though he were an intrusive hen. But when the intruder refuses to be dislodged, when the blood moves more slowly and the eyes grow dimmer, then it is that Dr. Winter is of more avail than all the drugs in his surgery. Dying folk cling to his hand as if the presence of his bulk and vigour gives them more courage to face the change; and that kindly, windbeaten face has been the last earthly impression which many a sufferer has carried into the unknown.[21]

The author and his colleague Patterson – young, up-to-date doctors – are disdainful of and secretly criticise Dr Winter, considering that the 'judicial frame of mind', rather than the sympathetic is the essential one. However when the author is stricken with a terrible bout of influenza with a splitting headache and pains in every joint, he muses:

It was of Patterson, naturally, that I thought, but somehow the idea of him had suddenly become repugnant to me. I thought of his cold, critical attitude, of his endless questions, of his tests and his tappings. I wanted something more soothing -- something more genial.

'Mrs. Hudson,' said I to my housekeeper, 'would you kindly run along to old Dr. Winter and tell him that I should be obliged to him if he would step round?'

She was back with an answer presently. 'Dr. Winter will come round in an hour or so, sir; but he has just been called in to attend Dr. Patterson.'[21]

In 1936, Chauncey Leake gave a talk to the General Medicine section of the California Medical Association.[22] He spoke about the 'problem of holding together for effective teamwork that spirited and often poorly harnessed pair, the scientific and the artistic phases of practice'. Until the time of his talk, he considered the art of medicine had predominated. However, he commented that now the 'scientific part of the team has almost run away with the wagon, and it is time to pull in the reins and get the team working together again'. Leake does not dispute the importance of science. For him, the artistic part of practice is the application of scientific knowledge to the patient's problem. Scientific data is reproducible, while the artistry of medical practice is down to the individual practitioner. Leake observes, 'Most of the science of medicine may be learned in the four years of medical school, but the rest of a physician's life may still find him deficient in the art.'

He elaborates:

> ...no musician, not even Beethoven, is a greater artist than the physician who develops a harmony of adjustment from the dissonances of a psychopathic personality; no painter not even a Romney, whose pink-cheeked maidens brighten every big gallery, is a greater artist than the physician who can put the bloom of good health in the cheeks of his patients; no dramatist or actor is a greater artist than the physician who daily plays his role in the everlasting and thrilling drama of the lives and deaths of his patients...All good physicians are good artists.[22]

'Gaudeamus', a poem, written and read by physician John Stone almost 50 years later at a USA medical graduation ceremony, encapsulates Leake's sentiments. He speaks about 'the arts' which are called by some 'soft data' when they are in reality the 'hard data' which is more relevant in life. He bewails doctors coming to a late awareness of the importance of the arts, training only to listen for the oboe in the whole orchestra instead of using the 'inner ear' to strain to hear the 'thin reed' of the patient's crying'.[23]

Scott Wright and others suggest 52 precepts that doctors and medical trainees should consider regularly.[24] These are some of them:

➤ listening
➤ showing the utmost respect for all patients
➤ being humanistic, compassionate and caring
➤ recognising the patient as teacher
➤ thinking about and planning how to best deliver the information before telling important news to patients about their health
➤ avoiding being cynical
➤ continually searching for meaning in medical work
➤ striving to achieve personal awareness and an understanding of personal beliefs, values and attitudes.

As well as striving to achieve an understanding of our beliefs, values and attitudes, I would say that it is equally important to understand the beliefs, values and attitudes of patients. Patients often draw on their religious beliefs at times of illness. The 'beneficent physician' who is committed to the patients' best interests must consider how best to support and respect patients' belief systems that may be helping them cope with illness. This is relevant even when the doctor does not have such belief systems.[25] It is also relevant when caring for children, as meeting the health needs of each child demands that healthcare professionals consider the cultural background, ethnicity, religious and health beliefs of the child and his or her family.[26]

Listening to voices

Scott Wright also recommends that a doctor should 'strive to be a healer'. Etymologically the word derives from 'hale' and means to 'make whole'. Doctors need to know how to listen to the 'thin reed' of a patient's crying in order to heal.
Frank points out

> one of our most difficult duties as human beings is to listen to the voices of those who suffer. The voices of the ill are easy to ignore, because these voices are often faltering in tone and mixed in message, particularly in their spoken form before some editor has rendered them fit for reading by the healthy…These voices bespeak conditions of embodiment that most of us would rather forget our own vulnerability to…in listening for the other, we listen for ourselves.[27]

It is important to listen to the voices of the ill before editing away what we regard as irrelevant or even uncomfortable. Healthcare professionals need to listen to and understand their patient's illness experience and be aware of their coping strategies.[10] One study found that African Americans used prayer to help them cope with health problems and bereavement.[28]

The 1989 joint working party report of the Royal College of General Practitioners (RCGP) and the Churches' Council for Health and Healing (CCHH) produced a publication entitled 'Whole person medicine – a Christian perspective'.[29] The Council and the College encouraged 'closer cooperation between general practitioners and ministers of religion in the day-to-day care of patients'.

Consequently, a survey of 228 British doctors explored the theoretical attitudes of GPs to the involvement of clergy with 20 specific concerns of patients. These are listed in Table 5.1,[30] as are the concerns and the number of GPs who welcomed clergy involvement. The list features much of what GPs see every day and includes chronic illness, physical disabilities and depression. However, this theoretical perception of the role of the clergy was not matched in practice as 43% made no referrals to clergy during one year of observation, while 44% made 1–6 referrals. There were various reasons why GPs did not refer patients to a minister:

➤ 69% responded that they felt that such patients would self-refer anyway
➤ 51% believed that non-religious patients would not like to see a minister
➤ 19% said the patients did not hold any religious beliefs
➤ 17% had never considered this option.

Barriers to spiritual assessment

Two hundred and thirty-one family doctors in Missouri, USA were sent a questionnaire and the response rate was good at 74%. Nearly all the respondents – 96% – believed that spiritual well-being is an important component in health and 58% thought that doctors should address the spiritual concerns of their patients. The most common spiritual issue discussed was fear of dying and less than 20% of the doctors examined spiritual issues in more than 10% of patient encounters. They attributed the following as barriers to their undertaking spiritual assessment:

➤ lack of time
➤ inadequate training on taking a spiritual history
➤ difficulty in identifying patients who wanted to discuss spiritual issues.[31]

Other barriers, which prevent doctors from supporting the spiritual health of their patients, are:

➤ many practice clinical medicine in a strict biomedical model and spiritual matters may seem less relevant
➤ the effect of the spiritual dimension on health is taught infrequently to doctors at undergraduate and postgraduate level
➤ the spiritual needs of patients may be complex and daunting and therefore discourage any involvement of the doctor[6]
➤ patients may sense the doctor is uninterested in or hostile to spiritual matters.

Some authors argue that the link demonstrated between spirituality and health is at times exaggerated.[32,33,34] Sloan and Bagiella dispute claims that religious involvement results in better health outcomes. In one study, they looked at all relevant English language articles in cardiovascular disease and hypertension for the year 2000. They identified 266 articles published in 2000 but felt that only 17% were relevant to claims of health benefits associated with religious involvement. Half of these articles were irrelevant to the claims of health benefits while the relevant ones had significant flaws in study design or they were misrepresented. The authors conclude there is little empirical evidence to suggest that religious involvement or activity is associated with favourable health outcomes. There are also ethical concerns that when doctors depart from areas of established expertise to promote a non-medical agenda, they 'abuse their status as professionals'. Sloan and Bagiella argue that taking into account spiritual factors and their health implications is one thing whereas 'taking them on as objects of interventions' is another.

The doctor is called to practise *Primum non nocere* (first do no harm) and an objection to linking spiritual activities to health is the danger of making moral judgements on patients.

TABLE 5.1 Number of respondents believing that the clergy could be of help in caring for patients' concerns. (Reproduced with the kind permission of the *British Journal of General Practice*, July 1990.)

Patients' concerns	Number (%) of GPs responding positively (n=228)
Terminal illness	225 (98.7)
Bereavement	223 (97.8)
Marriage	215 (94.3)
Chronic illness	214 (93.9)
Divorce	214 (93.9)
Attempted suicide	205 (89.9)
Depression	200 (87.7)
Physical disabilities	195 (85.5)
Alcohol/drug dependence	193 (84.7)
AIDS	192 (84.2)
Big disappointment	184 (80.7)
Abortion	182 (79.8)
Getting older	182 (79.8)
Major accident	174 (76.3)
Unemployment/retirement	173 (75.9)
Infertility	154 (67.5)
Major surgical operation	152 (66.7)
New employment	118 (51.7)
Childbirth	114 (50.0)
Going on the 'pill'	103 (45.2)

Attempts to link religious and spiritual activities to health are reminiscent of the now discredited research suggesting that different ethnic groups show differing levels of moral probity, intelligence, or other measures of social worth.[34]

Patients could thus be given the unwelcome burden of feeling that their illness was due to their own shortcomings. Sloan and Bagiella are also especially critical of studies of the intercessory prayer genre and the inference that doctors should be prescribing religious activities. Byrd's study is one such example. Over a period of ten months, 393 patients admitted to a San Francisco coronary care unit were randomised to an intercessory prayer group or to a control group. The patients did not know to which group they had been allocated. The first group received intercessory prayer by study participants praying outside the hospital while the control group did not. Byrd found the control patients required ventilator assistance, antibiotics and diuretics more often than the intercessory prayer group. For him the data suggested that intercessory prayer to God has a beneficial therapeutic effect in patients admitted to the coronary care unit.[35]

Despite being uneasy with the conclusions that Byrd's and similar studies draw about recommending prayer, Sloan and Bagiella nonetheless recognise that no one can object to 'respectful support' for patients who draw on religious faith during times of illness.

Doctors may be reluctant to address spiritual health because of concerns about proselytising or they may feel that this area is the province of the patient alone. In the past, doctors had similar reservations about substance abuse, sexual history and other sensitive matters. These subjects are now discussed openly because of the recognition of their impact on health. The spiritual history informs the doctor of the significance of the spiritual dimension in the patient's life and the support that this could give in chronic, severe or terminal illness. A survey of over a thousand psychiatrists and physicians showed the former were more likely than the latter to acknowledge the positive influences of the spiritual dimension on health but they were also more aware of spiritual distress. The psychiatrists also appeared to be more comfortable then their colleagues in addressing this issue (93% compared with 53%).[36]

RECOGNISING SPIRITUAL DISTRESS

The purpose of taking the spiritual history is not to propose that patients follow a particular spiritual path but rather to discern if there is underlying spiritual distress, which may be making an impact on the patient's illness, colouring his presentation or enhancing his suffering. Spiritual distress may generate symptoms. In some patients, spiritual issues will not just walk away.

The Hospice and Palliative Nurses Association lists the following as signs and symptoms of spiritual distress in the patient:

➤ questioning of the meaning of life
➤ fear of falling asleep at night or other fears
➤ anger at God/higher power
➤ questioning of own belief system
➤ sensation of emptiness and loss of direction
➤ talking about feeling abandoned by God/higher power
➤ search for spiritual help
➤ questioning of meaning of suffering
➤ pain and other physical symptoms may be expressions of spiritual distress.[37]

Faced with illness we ask questions: Why me? What will happen? Will I die? What does it mean? We are also afraid.

'Third Generation'[38] is a tale by Sir Arthur Conan Doyle about congenital syphilis. It reflects the medical understanding of the time that the disease was transmitted via the sperm of the father. If left untreated, syphilis can damage the heart, nervous system, eyes, brain, bones and skin. The condition has a dreadful stigma attached to it.

Sir Francis Norton, a young baronet, comes to see an eminent doctor. That morning he had noticed a suspicious rash on his shin and he was terrified:

> He was a pitiful, half-tragic and half-grotesque figure, as he stood with one trouser leg rolled to the knee, and that ever-present horror still lurking in his eyes...

The doctor examines the young man's teeth and eyes, exhibiting a 'glowing pleasure' as he hits on the diagnosis:

> 'This is very typical – very typical indeed…Curiously enough, I am writing a monograph upon the subject. It is singular that you should have been able to furnish so well-marked a case.' He had so forgotten the patient in his symptom, that he had assumed an almost congratulatory air towards its possessor. He reverted to human sympathy again, as his patient asked for particulars...

At this point, the distinguished doctor diagnoses syphilis and the young man is very shocked at this discovery although he had suspected it – his father had worn gloves and had a similar rash when he was alive. The father had lived a quiet life while his grandfather's life had been dissolute and debauched:

> 'But where is the justice of it, doctor?' cried the young man…'The coarse and animal is abhorrent to me…And now that this vile, loathsome thing – ach, I am polluted to the marrow, soaked in abomination! And why? Haven't I a right to ask why? Did I do it? Was it my fault? Could I help being born? And look at me now,

blighted and blasted, just as life was at its sweetest. Talk about the sins of the father – how about the sins of the Creator?' He shook his two clinched hands in the air – the poor impotent atom with his pinpoint of brain caught in the whirl of the infinite.

The baronet was due to be married within a couple of days and asked if he could go ahead with the wedding. The doctor advised him to call it off but Sir Francis could not bear subjecting his fiancée to the inevitable public disgrace. He then left, promising that he would return the next day:

> Dr. Horace Selby heard again of his patient next morning, and rather earlier than he had expected. A paragraph in the *Daily News* caused him to push away his breakfast untasted, and turned him sick and faint while he read it. 'A Deplorable Accident,' it was headed, and it ran in this way:
>   About eleven o'clock last night a young man was observed while endeavouring to get out of the way of a hansom to slip and fall under the wheels of a heavy, two-horse dray. On being picked up his injuries were found to be of the most shocking character, and he expired while being conveyed to the hospital.

From our earliest years until the mysterious instant of death, suffering touches our life. It is part of our personal identity. Suffering has the potential to reveal a different world to us and to teach us something new. Yet suffering can also oppress us, make us bitter and harden our hearts. Suffering can cause despair. Suffering can break us or forge us. If we do not search for some sort of meaning, it is difficult to face the darkness of suffering.[39] We end up asking repeatedly why we suffer. Illness can be the cause of tremendous suffering and suffering can lead to spiritual distress.

FEATURES OF SPIRITUAL DISTRESS

The Hospice and Palliative Nurses Association in the USA defines spiritual distress as 'a disruption in one's belief or value system. It affects a person's entire being. It shakes the basic beliefs of one's life.'[37]

The nearness of death may trigger the need for connection, hope and purpose. Fear, despair, the feeling of isolation and uselessness may be pointers to underlying spiritual need.[40] Unmet spiritual needs increase spiritual distress and thus intensify the experience of illness or dying. Some clinicians,[40, 41, 42] believe that recognising the spiritual dimension of the human experience broadens the avenues of compassionate medical care whatever the patient's culture or the presence/absence of religion. Doctors may tune into to their patients' spiritual needs, be attentive to the possibility of spiritual distress, and prepared to respond with empathy.

According to Kliewer and Saultz, a person may move back and forth between spiritual 'stability' and spiritual distress. The characteristics of spiritual stability are:

➤ hope
➤ empowerment
➤ release/forgiveness
➤ restoration/blessing
➤ connectedness and serenity.

The opposing features of spiritual distress are respectively:

➤ despair
➤ helplessness
➤ anger
➤ guilt/curse
➤ disconnection and fear.[12]

Patients may communicate their spiritual distress through symptoms and signs such as withdrawal, anxiety, denial, apathy, anger, irritability, emotional distress and difficulty sleeping. The important thing for the healthcare practitioner is not to reach immediately for an antidepressant or hypnotic or worse subtly choose to pretend the problem is not there. We have to recognise the patient may be suffering spiritually.

Despair

Despair is the absence of hope. There is nothing worse for a patient – for any-one – than to feel there is nothing left for him: no glimmer of hope, nothing to look forward to or grasp. Despair is linked to meaning. If there is no meaning, why hope? There may be questions about the meaning of suffering and of exist-ence itself. Hitherto deeply held belief systems may topple when faced with a stroke, depression, failing vision, deafness…

Beethoven's despair is evident in the letter that he wrote to a trusted friend:

> To give you some idea of my extraordinary deafness, I must tell you that in the theatre I am obliged to lean close up against the orchestra in order to understand the actors, and when a little way off I hear none of the high notes of instruments or singers. It is most astonishing that in conversation some people never seem to observe this; being subject to fits of absence, they attribute it to that cause…Heaven alone knows how it is to end!…How often have I cursed my exist-ence! Plutarch led me to resignation. I shall strive if possible to set Fate at defiance, although there must be moments in my life when I cannot fail to be the most unhappy of God's creatures.[43]

Many who despair drag their feet along hospital corridors or sit unobtrusively awaiting their turn at a doctor's surgery. Despair wears many faces – its mask may be impenetrable. Despairing people often feel helpless.

Helplessness

Helplessness is a common finding when there is spiritual distress. In *North and South*,[44] 19-year-old Bessy Higgins has spent her life working in the cotton mills. She lives in Milton, a fictional industrial town in the North of England. She acquires a chronic respiratory disorder because of exposure to 'fluff' in the factory and suffers from coughing and shortness of breath. Her symptoms are an enormous burden and nothing is available to relieve them. She speaks to Margaret, the heroine of the book, about her plight.

> 'I'm better in not being torn to pieces by coughing o'nights, but I'm weary and tired o' Milton, and longing to get away to the land o' Beulah;[†] and when I think I'm farther and farther off, my heart sinks, and I'm no better; I'm worse.' Margaret turned round to walk alongside of the girl in her feeble progress homeward. But for a minute or two she did not speak. At last she said in a low voice, 'Bessy, do you wish to die?' For she shrank from death herself, with all the clinging to life so natural to the young and healthy.
>
> Bessy was silent in her turn for a minute or two. Then she replied, 'If yo'd led the life I have, and getten as weary of it as I have, and thought at times, 'maybe it'll last for fifty or sixty years – it does wi' some,' – and got dizzy and dazed, and sick, as each of them sixty years seemed to spin about me, and mock me with its length of hours and minutes, and endless bits o' time – oh, wench! I tell thee thou'd been glad enough when th'doctor said he feared thou'd never see another winter.'

Bessy is so tired that she believes she would be unable to enjoy heaven without resting first. One of the main sources of her pain is her father's atheism. She does not believe his assertions that the only reality is what can be seen and touched, however at night she is tempted to think that her life has no purpose and her suffering is futile:

> 'I wish father would not speak as he does...But yo'see, though I don't believe him a bit by day, yet by night – when I'm in a fever, half-asleep and half-awake – it comes back upon me – oh! so bad! And I think, if this should be th'end of all, and if all I've been born for is just to work my heart and my life away, and to sicken i'this dree place, wi' them mill-noises in my ears for ever, until I could

---

[†]Land where pilgrims tarry before they enter heaven.

scream out for them to stop, and let me have a little piece o' quiet – and wi' the fluff filling my lungs, until I thirst to death for one long deep breath o' the clear air yo' speak on – and my mother gone, and I never able to tell her again how I loved her, and o' all my troubles – I think if this life is th'end, and that there's no God to wipe away all tears from all eyes – yo' wench, yo'!' said she, sitting up, and clutching violently, almost fiercely, at Margaret's hand, 'I could go mad, and kill yo', I could.'

In Kim Dayton's short story 'Procedures',[45] the doctor/nurse-patient relationship goes horribly wrong. There is in fact no relationship. Mrs Colson wants only to see and hold her newborn baby. She is told that this is not possible:

> 'It's kind of like a fish out of water,' said the doctor, who was not really a doctor yet.
> 'What do you mean, a fish?' I asked.
> 'Well, what I mean is, do you know how a fish can't breathe when it's out of the water? Well, the baby has a similar problem.'

Mrs Colson hears that the baby has a device to assist breathing and some 'additional tubes'. She asks if she can hold her baby but is told again that this is impossible because of the 'standard nursery procedures'. She is advised to 'get some rest'. Later when she asks to see her baby, access is again denied because of 'procedures'. After some rest and while she is dutifully 'scrubbing' prior to seeing the baby, a different nurse approaches her and explains that she cannot come in because of the doctors' rounds. She continues to ask at further intervals to see her baby and each time meets rebuttal. She is encouraged instead to express her breast milk. Exasperated, after two days she sees the baby and is doubtful that it is hers. She can only think about its resemblance to an inert, immobile fish.

Mrs Colson is sent away because of further procedures and waits for a long time until she eventually falls asleep. When she wakes, she goes over to the window but cannot see her baby because of the crowd of doctors and nurses around the incubator. She starts to scrub, but then a nurse approaches her to inform her that her baby has died. She is finally invited to hold the baby.

In their business, the medical and nursing staff is oblivious to a mother's distress and her sense of helplessness. Absorbed in medical, nursing and clinical procedures they fail to hear the mother's silent scream. They do not take the time even to find out about her and put together the clues in her case: they miss the fact that she is unmarried (she is repeatedly called 'Mrs') and has no supporting partner, she has been thrown out of her home and she is alone to face this crisis. The task of breaking the difficult news about the baby is 'relegated' to a medical student – *'the doctor, who was not really a doctor yet.'*

Anger

Anger may be directed at the healthcare staff, the patient's relatives, the doctor, religious representatives, against God and even against the patient himself. Dylan Thomas watched his father – formerly in the army – grow weak and frail with old age. Thomas exhorts him not to leave this earth without a fight and to 'rage, rage against the dying of the light'.[46] Perhaps the poet is mirroring the anger, which his father feels. Perhaps he perceives that his father is resigned to die and experiences the anger that *he* feels he should experience.

Ivor Gurney, born in Gloucester 1890, is commemorated as a war poet. He died when he was only 47. He suffered from bipolar depression and spent much of the latter part of his life in a psychiatric hospital. He wrote the poem 'To God' while he was there. It expresses his sense of powerlessness, frustration and deep anger. This is an extract:

> Why have you made life so intolerable
> And set me between four walls...
>
> ...And I am merely crying and trembling in heart
> For death, and cannot get it. And gone out is part
> Of sanity. And there is dreadful hell within me
>
> ...And dreadful is the indrawing or out-breathing of breath
> Because of the intolerable insults put on my whole soul
> Of the soul loathed, loathed, loathed of the soul.
> Gone out every bright thing from my mind.[47]

Guilt, curse

There may be self-blame: what did I do to get into this state? What have I done wrong to deserve a 'punishment' like this? Guilt itself may cause symptoms.

In Chekhov's 'The Doctor's Visit', Liza Lyalikov suffers from attacks of palpitations. Dr Korolyov is called to see her and astutely discerns the cause of Liza's problem is not physical but spiritual. Liza's disturbed conscience and the resultant spiritual distress cause palpitations. She is the owner of a large factory, which somehow has demonic associations for her. It is a factory where Korolyov reflects that up to two thousand people work in harsh, nightmarish conditions:

> a hundred people act as overseers, and the whole life of that hundred is spent in imposing fines, in abuse, in injustice, and only two or three so called owners enjoy the profits, though they don't work at all, and despise the wretched cotton.[48]

Only once Korolyov moves from his position of scepticism to sympathy does Liza begin to open. Liza herself concedes that she is 'weary and frightened' and offers her own opinion that she has no illness. She goes on to say:

> I am lonely. I have a mother; I love her, but, all the same, I am lonely. That's how it happens to be...Lonely people read a great deal, but say little and hear little. Life for them is mysterious; they are mystics and often see the devil where he is not.[48]

Lisa reads during the day but at night, her mind is empty and invaded by shadows. Her conscience is troubled because according to her perception she is an heiress of ill-deserved riches. The doctor sees a resolution to her problem in giving up the factory – the 'devil' which bellows out each night.

Disconnection

Patients may feel totally cut off from their belief systems. They may feel cut off from the rest of the world and – if they are religious – they may feel cut off from God.

Tolstoy's *The Death of Ivan Ilych*,[49] is about a successful judge who has climbed the career ladder and ingratiated himself with society. Suddenly terminal illness strikes him. He shows all the above-mentioned elements of spiritual distress. He particularly feels anger, disconnection and fear. Within the disconnection and fear, he experiences immense pain – physical and spiritual. The world outside interprets Ilych's moans as torment from physical pain. No one imagines the spiritual distress that torments him. With the benefit of being able to see 'inside' him, the reader finds Ilych's fear and disconnection palpable. Ilych is disconnected from time, his doctor, family, society.

...from time. Ivan Ilych is disconnected from time:

> Whether it was morning or evening, Friday or Sunday, made no difference, it was all just the same: the gnawing, unmitigated, agonizing pain, never ceasing for an instant...

...from medicine. Ilych is disconnected from his medicine. He takes it unconvinced that it will give him relief:

> 'No, it won't help. It's all tomfoolery, all deception,' he decided as soon as he became aware of the familiar, sickly, hopeless taste.

...from the doctor. Ivan Ilych does not trust his doctor and he does not feel that he has a sincere relationship with him. The doctor adopts a forced persona that is completely out of place with what his patient is experiencing. Ilych is disconnected from his physician, the physician is also disconnected from him. The doctor does not seem to recognise Ilych's real pain, adopts initially a playful attitude and goes through what Ilych perceives to be the ritual of examination:

> Ivan Ilych knows quite well and definitely that all this is nonsense and pure deception, but when the doctor, getting down on his knee, leans over him, putting his ear first higher then lower, and performs various gymnastic movements over him with a significant expression on his face, Ivan Ilych submits to it all as he used to submit to the speeches of the lawyers, though he knew very well that they were all lying and why they were lying.

...from wife and family. Ilych feels that just as the doctor had adopted a particular attitude, which he could not abandon, towards him, so his wife had formed one too – that he was not doing something that he ought to and that he himself was to blame though she reproached him lovingly for this. Instead, Ilych feels intense animosity towards her:

> Ivan Ilych looks at her, scans her all over, sets against her the whiteness and plumpness and cleanness of her hands and neck, the gloss of her hair, and the sparkle of her vivacious eyes. He hates her with his whole soul. And the thrill of hatred he feels for her makes him suffer from her touch.

There is a description of a family scene. Ilych's wife, children and future son-in-law pass by to greet him before going to the theatre to see Sarah Bernhardt the internationally acclaimed actress. However, they themselves are the unwitting actors in another drama. Ilych himself has insisted the family go to the theatre but he still feels angry. His daughter has what he will never have again – health and vigour. She comes in evening dress, 'evidently in love, and impatient with illness, suffering, and death' because they disturb her happiness. He does not connect with his son who is deeply upset and pities his father. The family tries to make conversation but speech breaks off when they realize that Ilych is staring at them with glittering, indignant eyes.

...from society. Although living in a crowded town, surrounded by many relatives and acquaintances, Ilych feels loneliness likened to being at the bottom of the sea or under the earth.

Fear...

...of being alone. At times Ivan Ilych dreads being alone and uses ploys to keep his servant with him:

> Peter went to the door, but Ivan Ilych dreaded being left alone. 'How can I keep him here? Oh yes, my medicine.'

...of altered physical appearance.

> And Ivan Ilych began to wash. With pauses for rest, he washed his hands and then his face, cleaned his teeth, brushed his hair, looked in the glass. He was terrified by what he saw…While his shirt was being changed he knew that he would be still more frightened at the sight of his body, so he avoided looking at it.

...of pain.

He fears his pain and its nature becomes increasingly evident. It is the pain of having lived a useless life. This spiritual pain is so much bound up with his physical pain that his carers have no idea of its existence. The morphine, which he is repeatedly given, lulls him into unconsciousness but he wakes to find the pain still there.

> But the pain, why this pain? If it would only cease just for a moment!' And he moaned...Left alone Ivan Ilych groaned not so much with pain, terrible though that was, as from mental anguish.

At a certain point he feels that he and his pain are being thrust into a deep, dark, bottomless sack. He weeps like a child because of his helplessness, his terrible loneliness, the cruelty of man, the cruelty of God, and the absence of God. He asks God why he torments him. He does not expect an answer, yet weeps because there is no response. Ilych then begins to listen to 'the voice of his soul'. The naked truth of his life is exposed and he questions its real meaning. He looks at the good-natured face of his servant and he suddenly asks himself, 'What if my whole life has been wrong?'

> It occurred to him that what had appeared perfectly impossible before, namely that he had not spent his life as he should have done, might after all be true.

When he has the courage and honesty to listen to the voice of his soul, he gradually judges his life critically and sees its futility. He wonders if the 'scarcely noticeable impulses which he had immediately suppressed' during his life might have been 'the real thing, and all the rest false'. In his family and the life that he had constructed all around him, he sees himself and all that he had lived for and he 'saw clearly that it was not real at all but a terrible and huge deception which had hidden both life and death'. This discovery intensifies his physical suffering tenfold and he groans and tosses about even more.

> From that moment the screaming began that continued for three days, and was so terrible that one could not hear it through two closed doors without horror…he realised that he was lost, that there was no return, that the end had come, the very end, and his doubts were still unsolved and remained doubts.

Once Ilych accepts his life and death, he no longer experiences pain or fear and in place of death, there is light.

THE HIDDEN AGENDA

Spiritual distress is not just isolated to serious illness but it may lie behind the 'simple' things that patients bring to their doctors. As in serious illness, such distress may cause anxiety and sleep disturbance, but it may also cause general malaise, loss of appetite and vague, non-specific symptoms. It could be dismissed as 'psychosomatic' and not taken seriously. Sometimes at the root, there may be deep spiritual suffering the patient does not even know how to begin to articulate.

The minor symptoms of a cold

Raj, a British Asian, seemed a confident, twenty-something successful career man. He gave some minor symptoms of a cold. I was a bit surprised at his coming because he did not seem to be unwell at all. I thought that he might simply need reassuring, so I made a point of examining him and told him that his symptoms should resolve in a few days. I looked into his eyes to check that he was 'reassured'. Instead, I saw that he was uneasy. I briefly asked questions to see if he was anxious or depressed but his answers and whole manner appeared to confirm that he was not – something that I had already thought myself.

I made a gentle movement to end the consultation but I could see hesitation on his part at picking up the cue. I waited. I did not need to wait long. He was probably wondering, 'Will I…?' 'Won't I…?' while I was preparing to ask if there was anything troubling him. He looked at me, saw it was 'safe' to proceed and then spoke about the two 'lives' he was leading. One was a continuation of the life that he had at university: clubbing, parties, films and fun. The other life at home was that of the eldest son in a religious family where smoking and drinking were not the norm. When he was with one set of friends he felt entirely comfortable and at home and the same when he went to visit his family hundreds of miles away. He respected and adhered to his religion. He also had a girlfriend who was not Asian. He was very fond of her and was convinced that his family would never accept her – so he kept quiet about her!

Then I understood that Raj's problems were not mainly physical or emotional, but he had a problem that was primarily spiritual. He was a young man whose religious tenets were deeply rooted into his culture and psyche and I imagined he felt 'schizophrenic'. I did not have any answers for Raj – I did not need to have any. I simply said that if I were in his position, I might find myself feeling torn between two worlds. This was enough for him. His eyes sparkled momentarily. He felt understood. Someone had recognised and articulated his suffering. Someone had given his suffering – ostensibly a 'cold' a name. He smiled at me gratefully and left.

I'm tired all the time

A common expression that doctors and nurses – especially in primary care – hear from their patients is 'I'm tired all the time'.

> Well I'm just tired all the time.
> *Since when?* After I had the termination.
> Don't get me wrong, I wanted to go through with it.
> My head knew I was doing the right thing.
> We didn't want to have a baby then.
> We hadn't planned one.
> *No, I'm not depressed and I haven't lost interest in things.*
> *No, I'm not anxious or anything like that.*
> I'm just tired all the time.
> I don't have any energy.
> *No, I don't have any regrets.*
> I knew that we were doing the right thing.
> Well my head knew I was doing the right thing –
> I don't know about emotionally.[50]

Rosie admitted later that she had felt very guilty about the termination although 'rationally' she thought she had made the best choice. She resented that her husband had not helped her make the decision (she had tried to interpret what she thought he wanted) and that this event was something in her life she could not share with her friends. We were able to talk about this guilt and – in the right moment – about its relationship with the abortion and the fatigue. Facing her feeling of guilt and the physical symptom that it was causing were important. The fatigue improved.

SPIRITUAL ASSESSMENT

If the spiritual dimension is so important, if the *soul matters*, then there is the challenge for all of us – patients, healthcare workers and carers – to ensure that we give due care to this area when appropriate.

Religion and healthcare

In the past, physical and spiritual care were linked together. The modern idea of the hospital originated in the fourth century AD when the Emperor Constantine converted to Christianity. Until that time, the person who suffered from disease was excluded from the community. Instead, the Christian tradition underlined the close connection of the sufferer to Christ, recognising how he ministered to the sick and healed their illnesses. Christians therefore established hospitals to look after the sick. In the fourth century, St Basil of Casesarea included a hospital in the religious foundation at Cappadocia and monks like St Benedict in the sixth century built an infirmitorium in their monasteries for the sick brothers. Although this became a model for the laity, the greater number of hospitals founded during the mediaeval period were monastic institutions. It is estimated the Benedictines founded more than 2,000 hospitals.

Arabic medicine boasts great figures such as Avicenna and it contributed greatly to medicine. It founded some principles in scientific medicine that we use today.

Nizami 'Arudi wrote *Chahar Maqala (Four Discourses)* in the twelfth century and he delineates the characteristics of the good doctor:

> The physician should be of tender disposition and wise nature, excelling in acumen, this being a nimbleness of mind in forming correct views, that is to say a rapid transition to the unknown from the known. And no physician can be of tender disposition if he fails to recognize the nobility of the human soul; nor of wise nature unless he is acquainted with Logic, nor can he excel in acumen unless he be strengthened by God's aid.[51]

The Arabs founded hospitals in Baghdad, Damascus and Cordoba, admitting patients irrespective of religious belief, race or social class.[52] The importance of the spiritual dimension in healthcare is evident in Islamic medicine from its foundation almost 1400 years ago. There was a hierarchy in classifying disease and spiritual disturbances were considered the most significant.[53]

Many centuries later in 1837 Florence Nightingale felt called by God to undertake a special mission. She did not understand which task until nine years later when she trained as a nurse. Her acute observations of the sick reveal their spiritual distress:

> I have mentioned the cruelty of letting him stare at a dead wall…But the long chronic case, who knows too well himself, and who has been told by his physician that he will never enter active life again, who feels that every month he has to give up something he could do the month before…How little the real sufferings of illness are known or understood. How little does anyone in good health fancy him or even herself into the life of a sick person.[54]

Drawing on centuries of caring for the sick, the Catholic Church through a multidisciplinary team has set out a charter for healthcare workers.[55] Many might feel that they can identify with some of its principles. The charter advocates that for the healthcare worker 'the sick person is never merely a clinical case' – an anonymous individual on whom to apply the fruit of his knowledge – 'but always a "sick person", towards whom he shows a sincere attitude of "sympathy", in the etymological sense of the term'. The charter reiterates that scientific expertise is not enough, but welcomes availability, attention, understanding, sharing, benevolence, patience and dialogue. It recognises that sickness and suffering are phenomena, which ask questions that go beyond medicine to the essence of the human condition in this world. Sickness and suffering 'are not experiences which affect only the physical substance of the human being, but they affect him in his entirety and in his somatic-spiritual unity'.

Every intervention on the human body touches not only the tissues, the organs and their functions, but it also involves the person himself at various levels. Consequently, one cannot isolate

> the technical problem posed by the treatment of a particular illness from the care that should be given to the person of the patient in all his dimensions. It is well to bear this in mind, particularly at a time when medical science is tending towards specialisation in every discipline.[56]

The challenge for healthcare workers is to have an awareness of the values and meanings that make sense of sickness and of their work and to make every individual clinical case a human encounter.

The philosophy of medical practice

Edmund Pellegrino has striven to outline a philosophy for medicine. Drawing from Pellegrino's work, Perkins argues 'in order to enter the experience of the patient as a person, the physician must be willing to transcend the surface of the patient's illness and become vulnerable in experiencing the suffering of this person'.[56] Using the Pellegrino healing-relationship model, Perkins outlines that the main focus of the patient-clinician relationship is the 'covenant of trust' between the two. The one is sick and searching for healing and hope while the other has promised to care and heal. According to Pellegrino, the outcome of the patient-clinician relationship is a beneficial healing action that restores health and wholeness. This relationship consists of three components.

1 The fact of illness: the patient's experience of illness.
2 The promise to care.
3 The act of healing.

The healing relationship leads to the

> spiritual, psychological and physical good of the person who has asked for healing, not just the biomedical good of the patient. In this relationship, the healer, bound to the sick person through beneficence and trust, also experiences affirmation of his own personhood. He too may come to an experience of vulnerability, suffering and healing in this encounter. When a clinician avoids any experience of the pain and suffering of the sick person, or is unwilling to encounter the other in

the fact of the illness, the development of a healing relationship is inhibited, and becomes merely a series of tasks and technical activities.[56]

However, healing or restoration to health is not always possible and if this is the case, amelioration of suffering, adaptation to chronic or terminal illness and effective coping become the goals.

Pellegrino argues that alternate models are challenging the covenant of trust – the traditional notion of the patient-doctor relationship.

➤ Contract model: here the doctor and patient are bound by a 'legal' contract where the doctor will only do what is 'spelled out'.

➤ Free market relationship: here the doctor is the 'supplier' and the patient the 'consumer' and the type of care given risks being driven by market forces.

➤ Doctor as mechanic: the predominant asset is technical competence; compassion and caring take second place.[57]

For Pellegrino, medicine cannot be practised in some sort of moral or ethical vacuum. He offers a virtue-based ethic for medicine, doctors and healthcare workers and considers 'honesty, justice, benevolence, humility and courage' virtues of the 'good physician'. Compassion is another important virtue. He comments that one of the criticisms levelled at doctors today is the 'perceived deficiency in compassion':

> A good physician does not just apply cognitive data from the medical literature to the particular patient by reason of a catalogue or 'cook-book' of indications. Rather, the good physician co-suffers with the patient.
> …Compassion is distinct from mercy, pity, empathy or sympathy…Compassion focusses on co-experiencing another's suffering. Compassion includes an ability to objectify what another person is feeling in symbolic form, that is, in our speech, our body language, and our participation in the 'story' of the other's illness…Competence must coexist with compassion. It is only when the physician uses technical information, without reference to the things that make *this* experience unique for *this* patient, that she can be noncompassionate.[57]

However, virtues are not confined only to the doctor. In the healing relationship, virtues develop in both the patient and the doctor.

Person–centred healthcare

Kitwood's work with dementia is relevant to all branches of medicine.[58] He argues that instead of separating the person from his or her pathology, we need to redress the balance so we recognise men and women with dementia in their full humanity. Consequently, we ought not to speak about person-with-

DEMENTIA, but PERSON-with-dementia. Similarly, using Kitwood's example, we could substitute PERSON-with-illness for person-with-ILLNESS.

There are three main areas of discourse where the term personhood is found – transcendence, ethics and social psychology. The term has a different meaning in each area although there is a shared basic concept. In transcendence, the person is an 'icon of God' and in the field of ethics, there is the principle of respect for persons. Social psychology emphasises the place of the individual in a social group.

Kitwood describes how he became aware of 'depersonalising tendencies' in his work with dementia. He uses the term 'malignant social psychology' to describe elements, which undermine the personhood of the PERSON-with-dementia. The disturbing thing is that the term 'malignant' does not imply evil intent on the part of the caregivers – far from it! Generally, caregivers do their work with kindness and good intent. The malignancy instead is 'part of our cultural inheritance'.

Kitwood claims that dementia is not simply a disease with progressive loss of function and the 'person' but rather it consists of the PERSON-with-dementia + the personality + the biography + physical health status + neurological impairment + social psychology. I would add that it also includes the cultural and spiritual dimensions of the person. Social malignant psychology causes untold spiritual distress.[58]

These are the features of malignant social psychology:

BOX 5.1 Features of malignant social psychology.

> **Infantilisation** – treating a person very patronisingly like an insensitive parent
>
> **Labelling** – using a category such as dementia (I would add heart failure, lung cancer) as the main basis for interacting with a person
>
> **Stigmatisation** – treating a person as if they were a diseased object, an alien or an outcast
>
> **Invalidation** – failing to acknowledge the subjective reality of a person's experience and feelings
>
> **Outpacing** – providing information, presenting choices, etc, at a rate too fast for a person to assimilate
>
> **Objectification** – treating a person as if they were a lump of dead matter

We would all recoil at the thought of a person with dementia being treated in such a way, however as Kitwood says, this 'malignant' behaviour is not intentional but cultural. Healthcare also comes with its own culture – we have to recognise this. This culture permeates the way healthcare workers act and the way we relate to patients. It can sideline patients, ignore their innermost suffering and banish it (by failing to acknowledging it) to the realms of insignificance. Nadia had treatment for breast cancer. I asked her how she had spent Christmas:

> Christmas was agony.
>
> They told me I had bone cancer and I thought that was my death knell. There was something wrong with the scan so they squeezed me into an urgent appointment. I had waited three and half hours and by the time it was my turn, the consultant had gone home so I saw his 'understudy'!
>
> I spent all Christmas asking myself if I would die. Four weeks later, they then told me that it wasn't cancer but *blood vessels*. But now they want to do a repeat scan although the first one was supposed to be just *blood vessels*. How do they know then that it's just *blood vessels*?
>
> What am I supposed to think?

The reality is that each of us comes with his or her own culture – his or her own behavioural and perceptual norms and terms of reference. A definition of culture is 'the totality of socially transmitted behavioural patterns, arts, beliefs, institutions, and all other products of human work and thought characteristic of a community or population.'[59] Healthcare workers have their own culture but so do patients. Researchers such as Klein contend that modern physicians are preoccupied with the diagnosis and treatment of disease viewed as abnormalities in the structure and function of the body organs and systems whereas patients in reality are actually suffering from illness – the human experience of sickness.

Similar degrees of disease pathology may generate different degrees of illness. The cultural elements that govern the perception, labelling, explanation and evaluation of the discomforting experience all affect illness – *and strongly*. Klein argues that the clinician's neglect of the patient's illness is partly responsible for poor compliance, patient and family dissatisfaction with professional healthcare and sub-standard clinical care.[60] The spiritual dimension is expressed through the patient's culture. To elicit the patient's perception and model of illness, Klein suggests asking questions such as 'What are the chief problems your sickness has caused you?' and 'What do you fear most about your sickness?' If the patient senses the doctor is genuinely interested, not only will the patient's model of illness be made apparent but possibly all the dimensions of illness – psychological, social and spiritual.

Deagle considers studying anthropology, sociology and psychology more relevant in General Practice than the study of neuro-anatomy and biomedical statistics.[58] The fact that the culture of the healthcare worker often differs from that of the patient's (differing belief systems, world-views, behavioural patterns, medical culture and ethnicity) demands that the former be proficient in the art of cross-cultural care in the widest sense of the term. It means that all dimensions of our patients are of interest – including the spiritual one – as they may be an important factor in understanding their illness and suffering:

> The art of cross-cultural care involves learning how to transcend one's own culture in order to form a positive therapeutic alliance with patients who are different from us.[61]

Deagle notes that such transcendence may be painful as we become aware of our own cultural 'glasses' and how they distort what we perceive to be reality. Similarly, entering the spiritual dimension of patients – when we are called to – makes us aware of our own spirituality and this too can be painful.

Culture and spirituality

A doctor describes how he learned – the hard way – about the importance of culture:[62]

> She was 56 and lying prone on the bed when I first saw her. The duty doctor had admitted her the night before with lower abdominal pain and suspected that she might have pelvic inflammatory disease. She felt that she had a mass in her abdomen, however all the investigations were normal. Relieved, I went to tell her the good news but she did not seem satisfied. Her pain improved greatly the next day, but she said that the mass had now moved and was creating pain in the left side of the back. Urine tests showed only the presence of a few inflammatory cells. I persisted in my explanation that there was no serious underlying problem but she still was not reassured. In fact, she asked me if I was going to operate on her. I tried to explain that surgery was not justified but she still was not reassured.
>
> The next day, the patient was almost screaming because of back pain. I was anxious that I had missed something very serious...such as tuberculosis of the spine. An X-ray was normal. She again asked if I were going to operate on her. She knew the mass was still there. I then had the inkling there was some part of the story that she had not told us: something that I had not asked...

The doctor was working in Africa and the woman had come from a rural village. It emerged that when the abdominal pain first started, she went to see a traditional healer. He said that she had been bewitched and had 'something moving' in her abdomen. The only way to get rid of it was to pay money to the traditional doctor or her ancestors would punish her. The woman was poor and could not afford to pay the traditional 'healer' immediately. She was spiritually distressed and the thing that was moving inside her began to increase her symptoms. A nurse was able to allay her fears and using metaphor that the patient could understand, explain that she could pay the money when it was available and that her ancestors would understand and would not punish her. The patient then became more relaxed when the doctor did his rounds later in the day. She stated that she did not have any pain and requested discharge. She was able to go home the next day, completely free of symptoms.

Kleinman and others maintain that cultural factors have to be considered in clinical practice as they surface as specific 'ethno-medical beliefs' (assumptions, expectations, interpretations, attitudes) that concern the body, its physiology and the self. Cultural factors may also determine perceptions about the causes and consequences of sickness, the search for therapy, treatment choice, compliance, satisfaction and many other issues.[63] However, clinicians similarly have their own cultural traits, which may facilitate or impede effective clinical care. Common sense would suggest that the wider the gap between patient and doctor, the more potential there is for difficulty. Ellis notes that cross-cultural difficulties are not just strictly ethnic as there are subcultures within cultures. Ultimately, almost all consultations are multicultural in some way.[64] There are differences in age, background, education, sex, occupation and vocabulary. There are also differences in religious practice, spiritual expression and world-view.

If we accept that culture is the totality of socially transmitted behavioural patterns, arts, beliefs, institutions, and all other products of human work and thought characteristic of a community or population, it follows that spirituality and culture are linked. Culture and spirituality are woven together. Sayings and proverbs are one of the main ways that African philosophy has been transmitted through the ages. They often have an educational role. For example, this proverb from the Baganda people of Uganda teaches the value of suffering:

> *Akutwala ekiro omusiima bukedde.* At dawn you will appreciate the one who forces you to travel at night.

It means that unavoidable suffering transforms the individual into a mature, responsible person fitting for society.[65]

This is another African proverb:

> Whoever does not suffer, weep or smile is not a man and whoever does not die is a god.[65]

Every culture also faces illness and death according to its own world-view. It is enough to think about the approach to illness of countries as diverse as Algeria and New Zealand. The religious dimension occupies a central place in many cultures and reveals the fundamental way that communities look at life and the world. Anthropological studies give religious belief central importance in the heart of every culture as it gives meaning to life and to events.[65] African culture is no exception:

> I've had the privilege of looking after people who were very ill and among them were the first cases of AIDS appearing in the hospital where I worked...I found myself with human beings who never doubted their personal wholeness even in terrible situations. I found myself face-to-face with someone in peace who, even though aware that anything could happen, still felt he was in 'good hands'...It was not the fatalism of one who resigns himself to an unknown overwhelming fate; not even an act of fatality, but rather a kind of confidence and trust in human, community and cosmic existence in which the most profound aspect of his being is inserted.
>
> ...In these moments the community surrounds the sick person; friends come to visit and no visitor is unwanted...It seems that the attention of the family is not really focussed on the mechanics of the illness or in the process of treatment, but rather on strengthening the vital link that has been weakened in the heart of the community. The illness is a sign, or symptom, of this weakness and every effort has to be taken to sustain the unstable social structure...Healing involves the whole community and not just the sick person.[65]

If you were to ask an African why we suffer, why there is pain and the meaning of sadness or joy and even why there is death, he would give a spiritual reason. He would tell you to ask God who made everything. It is usual to think that a person suffers because he has broken his relationship between himself and other people, between himself and the world, between himself and his ancestors, between himself and God.[65]

The phenomenon of atheism is generally confined to the West. Indeed the French philosopher, André Glucksmann asks the reason why Europe is the only continent in the whole world and in humanity's history to produce a civilisation without God.[66] Atheism however is not the experience of much of the world's population. In fact, if the world were reduced to a village of 1000 people, there would be 300 Christians, 175 Muslims, 128 Hindus, 55 Buddhists, 47 Animists and 210 of other or no religion.[67] The world is becoming increasingly smaller with migration, mass media and travel. People bring with them their cultures, religions and world-views. A serious illness may remind a Buddhist of the need to transcend desire and attachment, a Muslim looks to the joys and comforts of the afterlife maintaining faith in God through all his pain while a Christian considers that suffering has been dignified because Christ suffered. Not everyone has a religious world-view. If healthcare is truly person-centred, we need to consider that for some patients – religious and non-religious – the spiritual dimension may be very important in their perception of illness.

HOW TO DO A SPIRITUAL ASSESSMENT

Squeezing yet something else into the medical consultation, given the limited contact time between the patient and any member of the healthcare team, could understandably meet resistance. However, the idea of doing a spiritual assessment is not to pander to 'political correctness', or fill in yet another list of tick-boxes. In fact, an increased awareness of the importance of the spiritual assessment does not mean that every patient needs one. Rather it means acquiring the same awareness that we have of the value of the family history, social history or occupational history.

Just as some clues in the patient might lead to our dwelling more on the family history because she has breast cancer or on the social history because she has come yet again with a black eye, similarly certain pointers may make us think more about doing a spiritual assessment. The obvious one is the nearness of death, but there are many other times when a patient might be suffering from spiritual distress. There might be the burden of a chronic illness, a recent bereavement or divorce, the presence of mental health problems, redundancy, unemployment, the life changes brought on by a diagnosis, the suspense of a blood test, frequent attendance at a doctor's surgery when there is little evidence of pathology...the list is endless. I suppose the key to thinking that the spiritual dimension might be playing a strong factor in an illness, is having the antennae to detect this and having compassion. If we 'suffer with' the patient, then we shall be able to feel the distress that the illness brings and imagine what the spiritual needs might be.

Certainly, performing a spiritual assessment requires that the doctors and nurses reflect deeply about their own spirituality – otherwise there is the risk of going to the patient without any tools to help him or her discern the type of help needed (for example referral to the chaplaincy team etc). Instead of addressing spiritual distress, the healthcare worker might attribute 'pain' to the disease and unintentionally cause more suffering as with Ivan Ilych.

It does not need to take a long time to do a spiritual assessment. We may detect that patients are spiritually distressed by looking into the eyes, observing the body language, picking up pointers, such as how they talk about their illness. Does there seem to be fear? What understanding do they have about their illness and its causation? What do they think would make it better? How do they cope from day-to-day? How would *I* cope in their situation? What resources might *I* need?

A few words may reveal intense suffering.

There is an anecdote that Ernest Hemmingway bet ten dollars that he could write an entire story in six words. Although these words were falsely attributed to him, they nevertheless tell a story:

For sale: baby shoes, never worn.

These six words conjure up this picture for me:

> It is the Great Depression. A woman sadly fingers a box of pink baby shoes. She has hoped year after year for a pregnancy that she knows now will never come. Reluctantly she waits now for an answer to the advertisement. Desperate for money, she is bitter at the cruelty of life.

Formal spiritual assessment tools

'Caring for the Spirit' is a document produced for the NHS by the South Yorkshire Workforce Development Confederation in November 2003. It is not only directed at the chaplaincy and spiritual healthcare workforce of the NHS, but there are also implications for anyone involved in healthcare.[68] The document states that holistic care includes care for the physical, social, psychological and spiritual dimensions of the person and that these contribute to the health of those we serve. It points out that spiritual healthcare is not just the preserve of chaplains because 'the spiritual dimension is often expressed through the humanity of care offered by many health professions'. The authors note that with the support of policy makers, managers and lead clinicians, chaplains and other members of the spiritual healthcare workforce, we will all be able to make a greater contribution to healthcare. The document further recognises that spiritual care 'addresses the dimensions of illness, disability, suffering and bereavement that go beyond the immediate and the physical'.

'Caring for the Spirit' underlines the need to increase in the healthcare staff of today and tomorrow the awareness, education and understanding of spirituality:

> Educating staff about spiritual healthcare will enable them to contribute of themselves as well as help to meet the spiritual needs of their patients.

The spiritual history may be introduced as part of the normal history taking process which healthcare professionals (particularly doctors and nurses) undertake when they meet patients. The NHS Chaplaincy collaboratives of the South West Strategic Health Authority suggests various methods of spiritual assessment[69] including the HOPE Questionnaire and the FICA spiritual assessment tool. The HOPE questionnaire asks about sources of hope and meaning, organised religion, personal spirituality and effects of these on medical care and end of life issues. Puchalski and Romer[70, 71] devised the FICA tool for taking a spiritual history. FICA is the acronym for Faith, Importance, Community and Address so it is quite easy to remember.

Faith. The patient is asked if he considers himself spiritual or religious. If the patient answers 'no', then the doctor might ask, 'What gives your life meaning?'

Importance. There are questions to ask such as: 'What importance does your faith or belief have in your life?' 'Have your beliefs influenced the way you take care of yourself and your illness?' 'What role do your beliefs play in regaining your health?'

Community. Here the doctor or nurse asks if the patient is part of a spiritual or religious community and tries to understand how supportive the patient finds this.

Address. The patient is asked directly how he or she would like the healthcare provider to address his spiritual dimension in the context of providing healthcare.

Some authors[6] suggest additional questions such as:

➤ what helps you get through tough times?
➤ to whom do you turn when you need support?
➤ what meaning does this illness have for you?
➤ what are your hopes, expectations and fears for the future?

The 'Spiritual Assessment in Clinical Practice' course[72] is an online multimedia guide designed to draw on the spiritual beliefs, values and practices which may be valuable in patients' responses to stress or illness. As well as showing the clinician how to use the FICA tool, it also aims to:

➤ give an understanding of the importance of spiritual assessment
➤ demonstrate basic communication skills for addressing spiritual issues and concerns
➤ show how to incorporate patients' spiritual beliefs and practices into treatment plans where appropriate
➤ illustrate how to respond to the potential challenges which may arise.[73]

Another assessment tool is the Herth Hope Index (*see* Table 5.2). The patient is invited to read twelve statements and to indicate to what extent he or she agrees or disagrees with them. The Herth Hope Index has been applied in various settings – both clinically and in research – in areas as diverse as HIV, Parkinson's disease, cancer and mental illness.[74, 75, 76, 77, 78, 79]

There is also the Spiritual Well-Being Scale (SWB scale) by Ray Paloutzian and Craig Ellison (*see* Table 5.3). The SWB scale consists of twenty questions. The odd numbers in the question assess religious well-being while the even numbered ones assess existential well-being. The negatively worded items are reversely scored. Each question is scored from one to six, the higher number representing more well-being. The SWB scale is not solely confined to the spiritual dimension, but it indicates well-being at a physical, mental and psychological level as well as assertiveness. There are no agreed norms for the scale. It has also been used in clinical and research settings.[80, 81, 82, 83]

Herth Hope Index

Listed in Table 5.2 are a number of statements. Read each statement and place an X in the box that describes how much you agree with that statement right now.

TABLE 5.2 Herth Hope Index. (Reproduced with the kind permission of Kaye Herth.)

	Strongly disagree	Disagree	Agree	Strongly disagree
1 I have a positive outlook toward life.	☐	☐	☐	☐
2 I have short and/or long range goals.	☐	☐	☐	☐
3 I feel all alone.	☐	☐	☐	☐
4 I can see possibilities in the midst of difficulties.	☐	☐	☐	☐
5 I have faith that gives me comfort.	☐	☐	☐	☐
6 I feel scared about my future.	☐	☐	☐	☐
7 I can recall happy/joyful times.	☐	☐	☐	☐
8 I have deep inner strength.	☐	☐	☐	☐
9 I am able to give and receive caring/love.	☐	☐	☐	☐
10 I have a sense of direction.	☐	☐	☐	☐
11 I believe that each day has potential.	☐	☐	☐	☐
12 I feel that my life has value and worth.	☐	☐	☐	☐

Spiritual Well–Being Scale

For each of the statements in Table 5.3 circle the choice that best indicates the extent of your agreement or disagreement as it best describes your personal experience.

TABLE 5.3 Spiritual Well-Being Scale. (Reproduced with the kind permission of Ray Paloutzian.)

SA = Strongly agree	MA = Moderately agree	A = Agree
D = Disagree	MD = Moderately disagree	SD = Strongly disagree

1   I don't find much satisfaction in my private prayer with God.   SA MA A D MD SD
2   I don't know who I am, where I came from, or where I am going.   SA MA A D MD SD
3   I believe that God loves me and cares for me.   SA MA A D MD SD
4   I believe that life is a positive experience.   SA MA A D MD SD
5   I believe that God is impersonal and not interested in my daily situations.   SA MA A D MD SD
6   I feel unsettled about my future.   SA MA A D MD SD

(continued)

TABLE 5.3 Spiritual Well-Being Scale (continued)

7	I have a personally meaningful relationship with God.	SA MA A D MD SD
8	I feel very fulfilled and satisfied with life.	SA MA A D MD SD
9	I don't get much personal strength and support from my God.	SA MA A D MD SD
10	I feel a sense of well-being about the direction my life is headed in.	SA MA A D MD SD
11	I believe that God is concerned about my problems.	SA MA A D MD SD
12	I don't enjoy much about life.	SA MA A D MD SD
13	I don't have a personally satisfying relationship with God.	SA MA A D MD SD
14	I do feel good about my future.	SA MA A D MD SD
15	My relationship with God helps me not to feel lonely.	SA MA A D MD SD
16	I feel that life is full of conflict and unhappiness.	SA MA A D MD SD
17	I feel most fulfilled when I'm in close communion with God.	SA MA A D MD SD
18	Life doesn't have much meaning.	SA MA A D MD SD
19	My relationship with God contributes to my sense of well-being.	SA MA A D MD SD
20	I believe there is some real purpose for my life.	SA MA A D MD SD

Charlton and others argue that in two studies they have found that both theism and atheism correlate with less depressive symptoms than the in-between state of existential uncertainty. Consequently, they have devised the existential conviction scale, which measures religiosity and existential conviction.[84]

SOUL MATTERS *MATTER*

Finally, patient narratives are a means of taking the spiritual history. Just simply asking the patient to share his or her story can reveal so much. Expressions such as 'I don't know what this is all about, doctor', 'I don't know what I believe in anymore', 'I'm afraid', 'I feel so alone!' or – more worrying – a failure to communicate amid what is obvious suffering, may reveal terrible spiritual distress.

In this chapter, I have tried to show the importance of considering the spiritual dimension in a PERSON-with-illness. Health professionals and carers may feel that they do not have the skills to do a spiritual assessment. They may not regard it as a priority. It might however be a priority for the patient, and spiritual distress the cause of mismanaged pain. Where there is spiritual distress, it is important to seek help wherever possible. Perhaps as doctors, therapists and nurses, this might be the only way that we can truly help a patient. Some years ago in a *Newsweek* article, a consultant psychiatrist said that excluding God from the psychiatric consultation is a 'form of malpractice' and spirituality 'shouldn't be left in the clinical closet'.[85] This is not just relevant to psychiatrists but at some point all healthcare workers in contact with patients may need to address 'soul matters'. Do we want or feel able to meet the challenge?

REFERENCES

1 The Bhopal Medical Appeal. Healing people takes a little money and a lot of love.
2 Woolf V. *The Moment and Other Essays*. New York: Harcourt Brace Jovanovich; 1948.
3 Azhar MZ, Varma SL. Religious psychotherapy as management of bereavement. *Acta Psychiatr Scand*. 1995; **91**(4): 233–5.
4 Harrison MO, Edwards CL, Koenig HG, *et al*. Religiosity/spirituality and pain in patients with sickle cell disease. *J Nerv Ment Dis*. 2005; **193**(4): 250–7.
5 Gowri A, Hight E. Spirituality and medical practice: using the HOPE questions as a practical tool for spiritual assessment. *Am Fam Physician*. 2001; **63**(1): 81–9.
6 Mueller PS, Plevak DJ, Rummans TA. Religious involvement, spirituality, and medicine: implications for clinical practice. *Mayo Clin Proc*. 2001; **76**(12): 1225–35.
7 Asser SM, Swan R. Child fatalities from religion-motivated medical neglect. *Pediatrics*. 1998; **101**(4 Pt 1): 625–9.
8 Fox K. *Watching the English: the hidden rules of English behaviour*. London: Hodder & Stoughton; 2005.
9 Eliot G. *Middlemarch*. 1872.
10 Barritt P. *Humanity in Healthcare. The Heart and Soul of Medicine*. Oxford: Radcliffe Publishing; 2005.
11 Klitzman R. *When Doctors Become Patients*. New York: Oxford University Press; 2008.
12 Kliewer SP, Saultz J. *Healthcare and Spirituality*. Oxford: Radcliffe Publishing; 2006.
13 Araujo V. 'The person in relationship: which reference?' Acts of the International Meeting: communication and relationships in medicine. Associazione Medicina, Dialogo, Communione: Rome; 16–17 February 2007.
14 Sontag S. *Illness as Metaphor*. London: Penguin; 1983.
15 Hebert RS, Jenckes MW, Ford DE, *et al*. Patient perspectives on spirituality and the patient-physician relationship. *J Gen Intern Med*. 2001; **16**(10): 685–92.
16 Ellis MR, Campbell JD. Patients' views about discussing spiritual issues with primary care physicians. *South Med J*. 2004; **97**(12): 1158–64.
17 Narayanasamy A. Spiritual coping mechanisms in chronic illness: a qualitative study. *Br J Nurs*. 2002; **11**(22): 1461–70. Review.
18 Buxton F. Spiritual distress and integrity in palliative and non-palliative patients. *Br J Nurs*. 2007; **16**(15): 920–4.
19 Porter EH. *Pollyanna*. New York: Burt; 1913.
20 Hodgson Burnett F. *The Secret Garden*. London: Heinemann; 1911.
21 Conan Doyle Sir A. 'Behind the Times'. *Round the Red Lamp. Being facts and fancies of medical life*. 1894.
22 Leake CD. Practica medici moderni. *Cal West Med*. 1936; **45**(6): 455–8.
23 Stone J. 'Gaudeamus'. *Music from Apartment 8: New and Selected Poems*. Baton Rouge: Louisiana State University Press; 2004.
24 Wright S, Hellman D, Ziegelstein C. 52 precepts that medical trainees and physicians should consider regularly. *Am J Med*. 2005; **118**(4): 435–8.
25 Puchalski CM, Larson DB, Post SG. Physicians and patient spirituality. *Ann Intern Med*. 2000; **133**(9): 748–9.

26 McSherry W, Smith J. How do children express their spiritual needs? *Paediatr Nurs.* 2007; **19**(3): 17–20.

27 Frank AW. *The Wounded Storyteller: body, illness and ethics.* Chicago: University of Chicago Press; 1997.

28 Ellison CG, Taylor RJ. Turning to prayer: social and situational antecedents of religious coping among African Americans. *Rev Religious Research.* **38**: 111–31.

29 Churches' Council for Health and Healing and the Royal College of General Practitioners. 'Whole person medicine – a Christian perspective'. London: Churches' Council for Health and Healing; 1989.

30 Jones AW. A survey of general practitioners' attitudes to the involvement of clergy in patient care. *Br J Gen Pract.* 1990; **40**(336): 280–3.

31 Ellis MR, Vinson DC, Ewigman B. Addressing spiritual concerns of patients: family physicians' attitudes and practices. *J Fam Pract.* 1999; **48**(2): 105–9.

32 Sloan RP, Bagiella E. Claims about religious involvement and health outcomes. *Ann Behav Med.* 2002; **24**(1): 14–21.

33 Sloan RP, Bagiella E. Spirituality and medical practice: a look at the evidence. *Am Fam Physician.* 2001; **63**(1): 33–4.

34 Sloan RP, Bagiella E, Powell T. Religion, spirituality, and medicine. *Lancet.* 1999; **353**(9153): 664–7. Review.

35 Byrd RC. Positive therapeutic effects of intercessory prayer in a coronary care unit population. *South Med J.* 1988; **81**(7): 826–9.

36 Curlin FA, Lawrence RE, Odell S, *et al.* Religion, spirituality, and medicine: psychiatrists' and other physicians' differing observations, interpretations, and clinical approaches. *Am J Psychiatry.* 2007; **164**(12): 1825–31.

37 Hospice and Palliative Nurses Association. Spiritual Distress. Patient/Family Teaching Sheets. www.hpna.org/DisplayPage.aspx?Title=Patient/Family%20Teaching%20Sheets accessed on 22 December 2008.

38 Conan Doyle Sir A. 'Third Generation'. *Round the Red Lamp. Being facts and fancies of medical life.* 1894.

39 De Beni M. *I Tesori Di Gibì e Doppiaw: educarsi alla relazione.* 2nd ed. Rome: Città Nuova Editrice; 2006.

40 Brown A, Whitney SN, Duff JD. The physician's role in the assessment and treatment of spiritual distress at the end of life. *Palliat Support Care.* 2006; 4(1): 81–9. Review.

41 Balboni TA, Vanderwerker LC, Block SD, *et al.* Religiousness and spiritual support among advanced cancer patients and associations with end-of-life treatment preferences and quality of life. *J Clin Oncol.* 2007; **25**(5): 555–60.

42 Chibnall JT, Videen SD, Duckro PN, *et al.* Psychosocial – spiritual correlates of death distress in patients with life-threatening medical conditions. *Palliat Med.* 2002; **16**(4): 331–8.

43 Beethoven L. 'Letter to Dr Franz Wegeler. Vienna, 29 June 1800'. *Beethoven's Letters 1790–1826, Volume 1.* Wallace Lady G, translator. 1866.

44 Gaskell E. *North and South.* First published in serial form 1854–1855 and in volume form in 1855.

45 Dayton K. 'Procedures'. In: Haddad AM, Brown KH, editors. *The Arduous Touch: women's voices in health care.* West Lafayette: Notabell Books, Purdue University Press; 1999.

46 Thomas D. 'Do not go gentle into that good night'. *The Nation's Favourite Poems.* London: BBC Worldwide; 1996.

47 Gurney I. 'To God'. In: Kavanagh PJ, editor. *Collected Poems*. Manchester: Carcanet Press; 2004.

48 Chekhov A. *The Lady with the Dog and other stories*. Garnet C, translator. Project Gutenberg [EBook 13415].

49 Tolstoy L. *The Death of Ivan Ilych*. Maude L and Maude A, translators. Oxford: Oxford University Press; 1971.

50 Aghadiuno M. 'I'm tired all the time'. Author's own.

51 Browne EG. *Revised Translation of the* Chahar Maqala (*Four Discourses*) *of Samarqand*. London: Cambridge University Press; 1921.

52 'Hospital'. Encyclopaedia Britannica. 2006.

53 Khan MS. *Islamic Medicine*. London: Routledge & Kegan Paul; 1986.

54 Nightingale F. *Notes on Nursing. What It Is And What It Is Not*. 1898.

55 Pontifical Council for Pastoral Assistance to Healthcare workers. Vatican City, 1995. www.vatican.edu/roman_curia/pontifical_councils/hlthwork/documents/rc_pc_hlthwork_doc_19950101_charter_en.html

56 Perkins I. The physician in the moment of grace. *Ethics Medics*. 2008; **33**(9): 2.

57 Pellegrino E, Thomasma C. *The Virtues in Medical Practice*. New York: Oxford University Press; 1994.

58 Kitwood T. *Dementia Reconsidered: the person comes first*. Maidenhead: Open University Press; 1997.

59 Reader's Digest. *Universal Dictionary*. Rev ed. Reader's Digest Year; 1992.

60 Klein A, Eisenberg L, Good B. Culture, illness and care: clinical lessons from anthropologic and cross-cultural research. *Focus*. 2006; **IV**(1): 140–9.

61 Deagle GL. The art of cross-cultural care. *Can. Fam. Physician*. 1986; **32**: 1315–17.

62 Di Mattia P. *Olismo: il futuro della medicina? Nuova Umanità*. 2003; **XXV**(3–4): 419–45.

63 Kent-Smith C, Kleinman A. Beyond the biomedical model: integration of psychosocial and cultural orientations. In: Taylor RB, editor. *Fundamentals of Family Medicine*. New York: Springer-Verlag; 1988.

64 Ellis C. Ukufa KwaBantu. *SA Family Practice*. 1996: 125–48.

65 Centro per l'inculturazione. *Sofferenza, malattia e morte nell'Africa sub-sahariana: prospettive per l'inculturazione*. Makuyu: Don Bosco Printing Press; 2005.

66 Glucksmann A. *La Trosième Mort de Dieu*. Paris: Nil Editions; 2000.

67 State of the Village Report. www.ppu.org.uk/learn/infodocs/pm_globalvillage.html (accessed 2 February 2009).

68 'Caring for the Spirit'. South Yorkshire Workface Development Confederation. 2003.

69 NHS Chaplaincy Collaboratives. Spiritual Assessment. www.nhs-chaplaincy-collaboratives.com/col_sw_ds_assesssmentmethod_070522.pdf (accessed 22 December 2008).

70 Puchalski C, Romer AL. Taking a spiritual history allows clinicians to understand patients more fully. *J Palliative Med*. 2000; **3**(1): 129–37.

71 Puchalski C. Spiritual assessment in clinical practice. *Psychiatr Ann*; 2006; **36**(3): 150.

72 www.gwumc.edu/gwish/ficacourse/out/main.html

73 George Washington Institute for Spirituality and Health. www.gwish.org

74 Benzein E, Berg A. The level of and relation between hope, hopelessness and fatigue in patients and family members in palliative care. *Palliat Med*. 2005; **19**(3): 234–40.

75 Corrigan P, McCorkle V, Schell V, *et al*. Religion and spirituality in the lives of people with serious mental illness. *Community Ment Health J*. 2003; **39**(6): 487–99.

76 Fowler S. Hope and a health-promoting lifestyle in persons with Parkinson's disease. *J Neuroscience Nurs.* 1997; **29**(2): 111–16.

77 Gibson L. Inter-relationships among sense of coherence, hope, and spiritual perspective of African-American and European-American breast cancer survivors. *Appl Nurs Res.* 2003; **16**(4): 236–44.

78 Harrison R. Spirituality and hope: nursing implications for people with HIV disease. *Holist Nurs Pract.* 1997; **12**(1): 9–16.

79 Touhy T. Nurturing hope and spirituality in the nursing home. *Holist Nurs Pract.* 2001; **15**(4): 259–64.

80 Bufford RK, Paloutzian RF, Ellison C. Norms for the Spiritual Well-Being Scale. *J Psychol Theol.* 1991; **19**(1): 56–70.

81 Paloutzian RF, Ellison CW. Loneliness, spiritual well-being and the quality of life. In: Peplau LA, Perlman D, editors. *Loneliness: a sourcebook of current theory, research and therapy.* New York: Wiley-Interscience; 1982: 224–37.

82 Ellison CW. Spiritual well-being: conceptualization and measurement. *J Psychol Theol.* 1983; **11**(4): 330–40.

83 Paloutzian RF. The SWB Scale in nursing research. *J Christ Nurs.* 2002; **19**(3): 16–19.

84 Riley J, Best S, Charlton BG. The Existential Conviction Scale (ECS). 2005. www.hedweb.com/bgcharlton/ecsq.html (accessed 19 December 2008).

85 Woodward KL. 'Talking to God'. *Newsweek.* 6 January 1992.

CHAPTER 6

Becoming better acquainted

'Suffering becomes beautiful when anyone bears great calamities with cheerfulness, not through insensibility but through greatness of mind.'

Aristotle

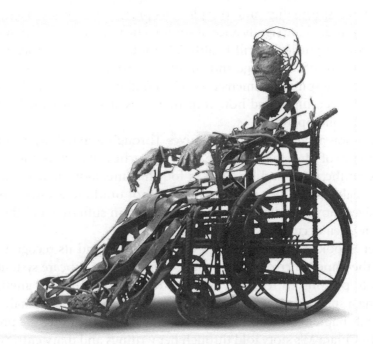

Agatha by Lau Hung

During my first years in General Practice, a good teacher said that whenever we discuss anything in medicine, we should ask ourselves the questions, *Who? Why? What? When? Where? How?* In writing this book, I think that I have tried to address these questions as far as they regard spirituality and health. I acknowledge that perhaps we have not journeyed in a linear fashion but proceeded as if we were on a spiralling staircase that seemed to go forwards and backwards and yet eventually reached the destination. This book is not about collating nice, neat data from investigations gathered carefully under controlled conditions in a laboratory but about observing people in the laboratory of life. The data therefore is raw and empirical but it is *living*.

Chapter 1 explored the meaning of holism and holistic healthcare. It showed that solely using a reductionist paradigm gives a partial view of the world, disease and illness. For example, interesting research in psychoneuroimmunology shows the limitations of the single-cause theory of illness and the interplay of stress and emotions in the onset of disease. This chapter also discussed the attraction of complementary medicine and the lessons that 'orthodox' health professionals might learn. It investigated the practical application of holistic healthcare as it embraces the physical, social, cultural, psychological and spiritual dimensions of the person.

Chapter 2 looked briefly at evidence for the existence of our spiritual dimension in the research of Sir Alister Hardy. It also considered the importance the world of education and the arts give to this aspect. There was an attempt to define the term 'spirituality' and to explore its place in the modern age.

Chapter 3 studied the significance of spiritual health and argued that neglecting this aspect might lead to ill health. We looked at spiritual health at the extreme phases of life – old age and childhood. Some space was given to the importance of the spiritual dimension and mental illness. A clinical case at the end of the chapter, illustrated how considering existential fears helps to treat patients with homeopathy.

Chapter 4 was all about patient narratives. Through storytelling, people share their experience of illness and speak of how it touches all parts of their humanity. They give the third and sometimes fourth dimension of what are often viewed in healthcare as two-dimensional – if not unidimensional – pictures. The narratives show the significance of spirituality in suffering and the central place that it often occupies.

Chapter 5 looked at the topic of spiritual distress and its recognition. We looked at the importance of spiritual assessment in a healthcare system where we advocate person-centred care. We also considered different methods of undertaking a spiritual assessment – some formal and some informal.

This final chapter is something of an appendix that illustrates the preceding chapters. In Chiara M's story told through her writings and diary entries, we see the importance of holistic healthcare. Formerly a nurse, she describes with crystal clarity the transformation that illness brings in her. Chiara's spiritual dimension is evident and its role crucial in helping her cope with her condition. It also explains the meaning of her suffering and existence. Chiara's story features in her books *Crudele, dolcissimo amore*[1] (Cruel, dearest love) and *Oscura, luminossima notte*[2] (Dark yet brightest night). I was so impressed when I read them that I wrote to her and asked her if I could translate and include extracts from the books in mine. She and her publishers generously agreed.

These words from a philosophy book encapsulate Chiara's journey through illness:

> True philosophy begins when someone awakens at a certain point in their life and discovers that he or she exists...Faced with this profound perception of one's own existence, we realise that everything experienced until then no longer has any meaning and no longer holds any attraction...It is like a new awakening to life – a life which our ears did not hear as we slept unaware of the clamour of the surrounding noise. We remember the questions that sometimes had occurred to us. We remember the answers (from parents, family and teachers) that made us think 'I exist because I must do this', 'I exist for that other person', and 'I exist in this or that sense.' Even if those answers are true, we now perceive an abyss between the questions posed by the realisation of our existence and those answers. These answers may have satisfied our intellect in some way but they do not explain this perception of our very existence. We feel the emptiness of former explanations...We sense a dichotomy between who we are and what we have known until now...This is when we begin to be true philosophers.
>
> There are two currents of philosophy. A true philosopher is not afraid of darkness, of problems, of the lack of peace. The philosopher abandons everything to seek truth by penetrating the darkness. He is then immediately faced with another choice: to feel that an Other is with him or that no Other is there. No philosophy exists which can avoid the choice of one of these paths. It is unavoidable – the choice of a Supreme Being or the choice of Nothingness. The philosopher enters a seemingly endless universe where he gasps for air, where there is no return and where he sees – perhaps – the faint glimmer of a far distant exit. Some people feel the presence of two eyes looking at them in the depths of the darkness. They do not see them clearly, but they walk nonetheless into the darkness, trying to find a link between who they are, what they seek to understand and that gaze which is more vaguely sensed than actually seen. And they feel the gaze follows them. They walk, solving their problems through the experience of coexisting with the Other. Some do not feel this gaze and walk alone. The darkness remains for both but with different outcomes.[3]

Chiara walks through the tunnel, sensing that Someone's gaze is always fixed on her.

CHIARA M'S STORY OF ILLNESS

> As you read the book, you have the feeling that Chiara's in-depth knowledge of suffering gives her the capacity to emanate this interior light. I read the book unable to put it down. When I got to the last page, I felt that I too had been on a purifying journey that made me see life from another perspective. It made me ashamed of not appreciating and loving it as deeply as she does.
>
> From the preface by Italian film director, Cinzia TH Torrini

A glance at the mirror

I look into the mirror and I don't recognise myself. Where has my face gone? Where did I lose it? I quickly draw my eyes away from the person who isn't me. I haven't managed to befriend it yet after these long years since the diagnosis. *It*. It has a strange name that they still don't know much about. A name that has the capacity to destroy you. Inside and out. I almost didn't feel anything at the beginning – just that terrible coldness in my hands – coldness that a pair of warm gloves won't budge. I was a bit ashamed of their marble to purple colour change. It wouldn't have bothered me but then those tiny, painful little ulcers broke out on my fingertips. One, two, three plasters that increased to ten until I looked like some clumsy cook who managed to slice her fingers instead of the vegetables. Then – I don't know how – I couldn't swallow a mouthful of that scrummy Gorgonzola cheese sandwich that I love so much. It stuck. I began to drink gallons of water each time I ate a pizza, a plate of rice or some meat. Then I began to differentiate between 'can do's' and 'can't do's' until I completely forget what I originally liked. I ended up just taking what would go down.

Then the pains began. Subtly…a bit at a time: my joints, muscles and tendons. I felt that I was a hundred years when I got up in the morning and I was jealous of my 73-year-old aunt who climbs the stairs like a young girl. I could not understand why my hands began to hurt too and why I could not bend my fingers properly. I could not stretch them out either and it was difficult to get a good grip with those plasters.

Now I get so nervous when I have to pay at the supermarket. I just cannot manage. So to get around the problem, I take out the paper money because at least when they give me the change I can open my purse and they can drop it in. Who cares if they make a mistake? Anyway, at the checkout they are all in a mad hurry.

The soft, velvety skin that I had before has begun to get hard. I feel as if I have been left soaking in starch. I have tried all sorts of creams. The shop assistants now start with the ones I have not used: 'Try this, it is the best moisturiser. Rose, Jojoba, Almond…' I would make loads if I were paid for recycling all the tubes.

However, it is my face – the face that I see and that others see – which is beginning to change. My skin is tight and smooth like a Venetian carnival mask. My lips are becoming so thin they are non-existent. I cannot manage to close my mouth properly and I am not comfortable with it. The only positive thing is that I will not wrinkle – just think of the fortune that people spend on face lifting!

To go back to my hands, they are wooden and hard. They're drawn back as if they're trying to grasp something that isn't there. The problem is when I'm introduced to someone: 'Pleased to meet you…' and I give my hand but…I'm completely mortified. They say that a man looks especially at a woman's face and hands. The annoying words 'beauty is skin-deep' don't convince me much.

An interesting case

At the beginning, the first hospital admissions were like a competition to see who could do more investigations. Blood samples or rather bloodletting. X-rays on all my bones, endoscopies, pH metres, ultrasounds of every organ, ECGs and EMGs. It is awfully painful when they put in all those needles that go deep into the muscles and give you an electric shock. Several biopsies on my body so they can look at the state of the connective tissue... The scars that I've got here and there are rather nice. Perhaps this could be the alternative to body piercing? There's always the novelty of a few 'experimental' investigations at each admission. And then those faces – so many – of trainee doctors who look at you and scrutinize you from behind the consultant. Then they politely ask: 'Can I feel? Can you show me? Open your hands! Lift up your head! Breathe deeply! Swallow!'

Each year it's always the same, if everything goes well...like a kind of car service. They say that I'm an 'interesting case'. OK, it's great to arouse interest, only I had meant to appeal to someone in a different kind of way. I have a sixth sense now. Shivers go down my spine when I see them coming, those white coats telling me: 'Let's go.' Endless hours spent waiting in corridors, summons, verdicts, proposals that leave me at a crossroads with some degree of risk. It seems like a detective story. I never know how it's going to end. And then many appointments. Too many requests to 'please undress' and each time I remove my blouse, they examine me, palpate every part of me with hands that are undoubtedly most professional but still alien to my skin. It's as if they're trying to extract some response that isn't there. I'm a defenceless, faceless heap. A potential store for medical discoveries.

And then the IVs (intravenous therapy). Finding a vein is like winning the jackpot. They have to warm up before they can get a needle into my skin. It never goes in first time... 'Try again. You'll be luckier next time.' I timidly try to point out the only microscopic, searchable area left but there's no guarantee I won't be faced with the obstinacy of someone who says: 'Don't worry'. Except that after riddling me with holes and leaving me with little purple memories, they end up going precisely to the spot that I had suggested before.

And then...the day comes when they tell me: 'We've tried everything we know, but don't worry, we'll find a solution sooner or later.'

That *is* consoling.

Taking stock...

I go home and take stock of the situation.

Physical tiredness is typical in this disease and I've had it since the beginning. It spreads inside too. I droop like an empty sack onto the chair – my mind a blank. I only have two options. Either I let myself drift off or...I lift up my head and get myself better.

Yes, but how? And what is my destination?

There is no place for me in this society that only wants 'good looks' as the first rule of its unwritten manual.

What can I do with my hands? And where can I put this coldness? I feel so different but what can I do? It makes me put off indefinitely invitations to go out until they stop coming. How can I explain that I can't drink and eat normally? If someone offers me something, I always reply with a smile: 'No thank you, I'm not hungry. No thank you, I've just had a drink.' Then I go home and raid the fridge to satisfy the hunger that I've felt for hours.

All my pursuits, aspirations, dreams and certainties wiped out by some sort of worm that little by little – metaphorically and literally – is gnawing right down to my marrow.

No!

A feeling of intense, lingering rebellion rises from the remnants of apparent tattered dignity. How does that song go? 'One in a thousand can do it...And why not you?'

Start again from scratch. Take stock of the past and the present.

Beginning with my face.

It's not my old face. I don't like it. I would be a masochist if I said I did, yet this is the face I have to live with.

And my hands? Before it was nicer to shake hands and convey warmth. I can't do that any longer. The challenge is to know how to convey this without them, if I find someone who accepts me and goes beyond...

Losing security for insecurity. But the thing that comes to the fore is what's essential in life.

I can't take anything for granted – not even getting through today. The vagaries of this illness are so remarkable that it still manages to surprise me although we have lived faithfully together for all these years.

Yet there's a sense of freedom and particular fullness in savouring the little, plain, insignificant and perhaps banal moments. They do exist, they are real, personal and they can become 'special'.

There are many things that I can no longer do and I am sure that others will be added to the list. However, I will discover to my surprise that there are many other things inside waiting to amaze me.

I glance at the mirror again. A tear courses down my smooth skin.

I let it roll – my dream fades far away...

This is my here and now.

> With my fragility and titanic strength.
> With my stubbornness and determination.
> With my tears and laughter.

With my will to find a way at all costs.
You need courage to live like this.
Lots of it.

Mere chance?

Emptiness, aridity, darkness, uncertainty. Just as the wind bears a fallen leaf on a faraway journey without a goal, so too You bear me in a constant whirling, falling, rising towards the only goal: God.

I wonder if misfortune is possibly hunting me down. Yet when I stop for a moment to reflect, I understand that this can't possibly be happening by chance. There must be Someone's hand behind all this...

Cheated

A month has gone by already. Mum is on the phone. She has been getting worse. She tells me that she isn't sure if she'll manage to hold out for me until Christmas. I put down the receiver and I'm in turmoil. Why is all of this happening? Who will give me back this lost time spent far from her? I feel my powerlessness and there is great rebellion stirring: 'It's not right!' I made a few phone calls to share what I was going through and I drew a lot of strength despite the pain that seemed to crush me.

If I could scream
If I could explode
If I could weep
I would.

Solitude

Alone with this silence
Alone with these thoughts
Alone with this suffering
Alone with these tears
That slowly trickle down my face.

Don't leave me

Don't leave me
When strength fails me
When I have no voice
When I cannot smile
When I will only be able to look into your eyes,
Please,
Don't be afraid,
Hold onto my hands,
But don't leave me.

Feeling understood

Here I am again in yet another hospital…

It (the illness) has put me through terrible moments. Moments where It seemed to have victory in its grasp. Many friends the world over have helped me with their thoughts, prayers, phone calls and letters. Yet there was a really tough time which I thought I wouldn't be able to get through. It seemed impossible. Luckily a special friend was nearby. She immediately understood there was no comforting me by sweetening the pill or by getting me to accept all this as heaven-sent… Not on your life!!! Don't say these things to someone who's doubled up in pain or plunged in total darkness! No – please – do not say them!!! They are not helpful. On the contrary, they make you more rebellious. If my friend had said anything like that I would have flung something at the wall.

Instead, she sat next to me, on the bed, she listened to me, she heard my despair, she gathered my tears, and her eyes looked straight into mine…almost as if she were physically entering *my* suffering, which in that moment became *hers*. She wasn't in a hurry to find ready-made answers. She listened to me right to the end…I could close my eyes…and feel that I was no longer afraid of the 'darkness'.

Like a candle

I feel as if I'm being consumed like a candle…

…sooner or later everything gives way. Perhaps I wouldn't have understood this without the illness – an illness which is 'detaching' me from my physical body and allowing me to draw out the inner spirit.

Crossing the bridge

I cannot refer to my illness directly. I have lived with *It* for years but they have never had a name for *It* – particularly when it comes to speaking to other people. We have studied each other sometimes through very hard struggles. There are visible, lasting traces of this battle. Every day *It* consumes a bit more of me. Every day the tiny muscles and minute particles of my body alter. It is gradual but unremitting disintegration. I am not used to it and I will never get used to it…

When they gave me a certificate stating the percentage of my disability, I understood that this was the end. Or rather, I had crossed the bridge that separates the world of the so-called healthy from that of the sick.

I tried for a long time to return at least halfway along the bridge so I could still feel I was in the world that I knew and didn't want to lose. At the same time, I was inexorably drawn into *another* world, still unknown to me but full of incredible surprises.

Droplet of light

All this grief and bereavement reminds me a little of the castle in the fantasy *NeverEnding Story*. The castle crumbles one piece at a time right to the end. Only a tiny droplet of light remains in the little princess's hand.

At the end of my life I would like to be a droplet of light (my essence) uniting to the Great Light.

Hidden jewel

When Michelangelo was working on marble sculptures he would say that everything was already inside...he only had to lift off the superfluity around it.

From an uncut diamond with Your golden chisel, You draw out the jewel that is in me (in each one of us) and that You have given me for safe keeping.

The present moment

During the last two years of living in obvious 'exile', I have had to live like that seed that falls to the ground and dies to give good fruit. It is like the darkness before the light, silence before music, winter before spring, and rest before motion. Who knows how and where I will be in two years, but the important thing is to live the MOMENT well, with the serenity of knowing the past is past and no one knows if the future will come.

Threatened immobility

Standing on the soles of my feet is agony. Moving from one side to the other or just getting up from the table to fetch a glass of water from the sink is becoming a mammoth undertaking for me... I got really frightened at one point, because the prospect of being in a wheelchair soon is looming over me...

No! I don't want to be resigned to this. I don't want to accept it. I don't want it.

They told me that I really would have to use a wheelchair if things go on like this. My whole being rebels against it. Why? A silent scream rips through my soul. There is only darkness ahead of me. An impossible future. I can't see anything. This ever increasing huge stumbling block is crushing me. Other people – those who can stand and move about as they wish – say: 'What choice do you have?! It is better than being shut up at home...It is hard in the beginning, but you will get used to it.'

To what? My God – get used to what?

I would love to be a pencil rubber so that I could erase this sea of suffering that people drown in, yet I realise that I can only discover the true face of each person I meet through suffering. Suffering annihilates, demoralises, destroys, wipes out security, and leaves you naked, defenceless and powerless.

But it purifies. This isn't mere cliché.

I can testify that it is true because I experience it day after day, month after month, year after year.

A drop of clear water methodically falls on a rock – heedless of the passage of time. Through its dogged perseverance it manages to mould and smooth down rock. It is just like this with people. Tears of suffering fall on the interior rock and they wash and hollow it out. They burn too because salt hurts wounds, but in that moment we are our true selves.

Pain

A foot ulcer has got worse. I can see the bone now. I can't put any weight on the soles of my feet even with slippers on... I cried non-stop, choking down the sighs so no one would hear me at this time of night as I sat on the edge of the bath with my feet soaked in water with antiseptic. I wept from the pain, power-lessness and discomfort. I cried out with my soul: 'Enough, I can't stand going on like this any more. I can't go on, let me end it now.' I begged my mother to come to take me home. I got angry with You and I even told You that I wanted nothing more to do with You.

...I never thought I would reach the point of having to tell You that I find it hard to live. But that's what it's like for me now.

Insomnia

It is eleven at night in this room all by myself in this incredible silence. I don't even have any thoughts. How strange...

I can't ask any questions and I don't have any answers.

Only this infinite solitude. A few phone calls, some comforting words that just add to this sense of isolation.

I am nothing – a nobody.

The future...what is in store for me? How much longer do I have?

Perhaps many people are thinking about me, but I am alone at this moment. Midnight.

Nothing. There is no way I can sleep tonight. My ulcers hurt...my ankle. It is not too intense but it is constant and annoying like a bee buzzing.

...I listen to the silence.

It is incredible. In a hospital ward at this hour. No noise, only the occasional sound of a car going by outside.

My soul is tormented.

What am I searching for? What can't I find?

Just as well, I am alone – otherwise I would disturb the person in the next bed.

Who knows if among the people I know, there is someone like me who just cannot sleep?

More pain

I have been in pain for seventeen hours since one this morning. Now instead of praying for a cure, I am tempted to pray for death.

Gleaning fragments

Another hospital, another appointment. Long hours waiting. The mingled smell of floor polish and disinfectant. Beds practically glued to each other. Smell of pain...inner revulsion, almost nausea. I would love to close my eyes so I no longer see suffering. As if simply lowering your eyelids would remove the problem! There's a story behind every patient, every bed and I'm gleaning only the fragments.

Night people

I like to think of 'night people'...People who are writers, poet, dreamers and researchers. Collective insomnia but in the positive sense. Who knows how much treasure lies buried in people who wait for the night for a bit of space. I'll also take advantage of these hours hoping the painkillers will work so I can think about that suggestion of writing a book.

But I am beginning to have my doubts.

What purpose will it serve? With all the books that exist, with the millions on millions of words spoken each day on the globe, why should I add mine?

Bright eyes

'I was already struck by your eyes on the train but this evening they speak. I've never seen eyes like them...I don't know – they have inner life, a special light...' [Comment of a girl whom Chiara met on the train.]

A smokescreen?

There are sometimes moments when I have a pressing need to question: 'And what if it were all a sham? What if what I believe in is just a smokescreen to avoid despair?' Luckily these flashes rarely come and attack the rational part of my mind....

Squarely matched

Something struck me today. I have to enter my suffering and not let it enter me...

On the surface, there doesn't seem to be any difference.

But I think – I know – there is.

We have to look each other in the eye – it and I – squarely matched.

In this way, I won't 'drag' it along and it will not crush me.

Suffering, who are you truly? What guise are you assuming?

Or rather – Who do you hide?

Rebellion

Watching a replay of my life, as if I were watching a film, makes rebellion stir in me. It stirs when I see the annihilation wrought by my vile enemy – this illness.

It is an exemplary worker. It is a perfectionist. It never takes a day off. It does not believe in holidays, convalescence or strikes. I cannot even plant a bomb in the house to 'blow It up' because we would both 'be blown up' together.

I want to rebel. But it is like wanting to demolish a rock-solid wall with your fists. It only ends up causing me more pain. Exhausted by the effort, I give in to walking by the wall until I end up crouched with my knees between my arms. I am dejected and completely powerless.

But YOU…Yes, I mean…YOU. Where are you?

What can You say to me in your defence? What sort of meaning can You give to my life?

I cannot take it any more.

I do not want to suffer any more.

This game between You and me is becoming too hard.

You have pushed me beyond the limit. I cannot go on.

The demigod

The 'Big Chief' or 'demigod' – as they call him – came today. In fact he has an aura of leadership about him (leadership in the negative sense). After I timidly asked for explanations and expressed my opinion about what I have been able to discover myself, he frowned, the other doctors in the group held their breath… (How dare a patient speak!) And he said, 'You stick to being a patient and we will think about everything else.' He turned on his heel indignantly and went away followed by a flapping, fearful swarm of white coats…

My head feels like ice. I have thousands of wild, rushing thoughts.

My first reaction: 'I will leave.'

The second: 'Why did I put up with it???'

I silently spend the afternoon hours looking into empty space or outside the window. My feelings vary: powerlessness, rage, frustration and longing…for what? For someone who sees me as a person, as a human being and not an 'interesting clinical case' or some piece that needs adjusting.

The inexorability of my situation sometimes makes me almost reconciled to my fate. Not in a resigned way – not this – but I'm reconciled in a realistic, fully conscious kind of way. If I share this with people, they are almost shocked and say, 'Don't say these things for heaven's sake! You have to fight, don't give up etc, etc.'

But do you know how long I have been fighting, how long I have been struggling not to give up? Why don't you try to be in my shoes for a week and see how you feel and then we will see…

Enough! I want to have the right at least to complain or to give my opinion without feeling guilty because I am not always looking on the bright side! I am not made of steel!

It is hard, so very hard. I never seem to come to the end of this long, dark tunnel…

It is true that many people are fond of me however sometimes they seem far away. It is like feeling I do not belong to any of them and the sense of loneliness increases.

If...

> If...if...if...
> If this were not that
> If the sea were not water
> If love were not joy
> If suffering were not weeping
> If my heart were not flesh...
> What would life become?

The wheelchair

From a letter to a friend.

...I knew the day would come. They did warn me about it, but stubborn as a mule, I tried to hide things and not draw attention to myself -as if I didn't have a care in the world. I did this for as long as I could, even though the pain was excruciating.

So you also know what happened. I went on to that notorious, despised wheelchair.

Everything rebelled inside me, like a silent scream with nowhere to go.

It seemed like the beginning of the end to me. I was convinced that I wouldn't have had the courage to go out and about like this any more. I know it might seem ridiculous, but I was mortified. The mere thought that people could see what I was reduced to gave me a constant, painful feeling of rejection and repugnance – something that normally shouldn't happen. I had even decided that I would remain closed within four walls for the rest of my life and only be seen by the people closest to me. I would be seen less and less in my own town.

I just couldn't manage to overcome it.

Then I was forced to go to an appointment in another town. I can't begin to describe the tension, the cold sweat that dripped down my spine and the strange positions that I adopted to hide my face. I could only see shoes and pavements. With my head bent, I didn't want to look the 'world' in the face. I felt exhausted at the end of the day...

...The first times I went out, at eye 'level' I would only meet the eyes of toddlers in their buggies. They were surprised at coming across someone with such strange dimensions in front of them. It's rare that an adult lowers down to toddler level, to the point that he can share a pram-ride! I felt awkward at the beginning. I could only see the negative side. I felt that I had in some way been 'demoted' in the eyes of the world. I couldn't wait to get back to my shell. But meanwhile an inner storm was raging...

A long ride by the lake with U and her friends.

This time it is different. Perhaps because I know that I am a stranger here, I feel brave enough to raise my head and look passers-by in the face. The day helps – the early hours of the afternoon, the mild air, the sunshine, the relaxed feeling. Naturally, the first ones are the children. I decide to be like them. To let myself be led…without a care in the world.

…We pause to have an ice cream. A woman emerges from the bar and smiles at me. I've made it. I have given you this long introduction to come back to those looks.

Remember what I was telling you about on the phone. Since keeping my head up, I have realised that people can look at one of 'us' in many different ways: curiosity (this really annoys me immensely, especially when it is morbid), embarrassment, questioning silence, awkwardness…

I have spent a lot of time thinking about this…

Perhaps…perhaps it also depends on us. What do I mean?

Help you to help us.

You do not know what to do and *we* do not have the courage to speak to you because we are convinced that we have been rejected from life by a world that rewards only activism, a career, health and an attractive appearance.

It is not easy being next to someone who is less able-bodied – no matter the disability. You instinctively withdraw into your shell so you do not increase the pain, so you do not feel the weight of the difference any more than you have to. You tend to meet, to look for a relationship with people like yourself and so unintentionally create – in some cases – real ghetto mentalities. But if I begin to say to you: 'Lucy, I need you. I need you to help me in this way…' I give you the opportunity to enter my world, to learn to know me and to speak to me quite normally.

Riches

I am beginning to realise the 'wealth' that this illness has given me. The capacity to listen, to enter people's hearts, tolerance, patience, the ability to begin again, to have no expectations…

Thoughts on death

As you have asked, I want to tell you something about death.

Firstly, I cannot bear it when people say the usual 'touch wood' and all the rest if I speak about it.

Secondly, the least they say is: 'Come on, don't think about these things. It will certainly come but not now!' Even when you are in hospital feeling unwell, you know the first ones to change the subject are doctors themselves.

I am not obsessed about it and isn't it obvious I instinctively think about life which I love immensely despite everything? It is only that as I am faced with a reality that is closer to death than life, I think it is right to be able to speak about it naturally, just like when you speak with your friends about a journey you're making. It is natural to do that, isn't it? You get organised. Oh dear, don't get the wrong end of the stick. I am not getting my coffin measured out! However, what is missing in these cases is discussion. Believe me, I have seen people suffer so much because in these moments they met evasive looks and half-finished sentences. They felt encircled by a desert because of attitudes like, 'I am not going to visit him because I do not know what to say.' Do you see? This kind of attitude is very common and it makes this turn of phrase even worse. I have had the 'privilege' to have a few 'practice-runs' and believe me, you learn many things. You learn to look at things with a sense of proportion, to see whomever and whatever is next to you in a different way. To be satisfied and adapt to things better, to feel time fly by as if its wings were brushing against your skin, to look around you as if you had been reborn and to rejoice in small, tiny things. Because of this, death does not frighten me. If anything, it is only that momentary passage, the uncertainty of not knowing 'how' it will be that frightens. But I believe that it will be all different, better and above all THERE WILL BE NO SUFFERING...

Chrysalis or butterfly?

I grope about in this painful darkness, a solitary figure – my soul in tears. A silent scream reaches beyond boundless galaxies and echoes repeatedly.

But where are you? Why don't you speak? What are you doing while I scream out my pain, my powerlessness, my solitude.

The lukewarm spring air, with the scent of newly sprung flowers, steals through the window.

Am I being reborn or am I dying? Am I about to be born again into endless darkness or am I dying in order to be truly reborn.

Where is my butterfly? Am I a chrysalis or a butterfly?

I would love to fly…away…far away…high up on a colourful, happy, sweet flight to infinity…to stretch out my wings and be caressed by the whispering wind of freedom.

But when will this happen? And at what price?

The value of suffering

'I cannot agree with you that 'suffering is useless…' In fact, I can say that I have become something of an expert in suffering – and not just physical suffering.

I have begun a course on exploring the unknown meanderings of my soul. Drop after drop, suffering hollows out the rock of my humanity. It gets rid of what seems indispensable, opens unknown doors of knowledge for me – doors that I would never have known how to find…

I do not want you to think that I am a masochist. Quite the opposite!

...You tell me that you no longer know how to pray. Instead, I am fortunate because I still can. Without God I wouldn't be able to write to you like this. Believe me, *Frà*, it is my last hope beyond all human resources.'

Silent scream

What do You think will become of me? What do you do with someone like me who does not understand anything at all? How on earth am I going to improve if for every step forward, I go ten backwards? Why do I not accept this illness? Why do I find myself so repulsive? Why do I still want to be 'normal'?

I find it painful to see myself like this. I find it painful that I cannot accept my own body. In fact, I have now realised that something else is happening to me. Sometimes I just couldn't care less. Not all the time. But when I notice them looking at me, I think, 'I'm a reject now. There is no way that I can get better. I shall always be labelled as "handicapped."'

Some people tell me not to think about certain things, but you know only too well that their reaction would be even worse if they were in my place. I would love to scream and release everything that is inside but I want to do it on my own, without other eyes or ears. And I cannot do it. This is awful.

Lessons

I have learned that you can:

➤ be silent without getting upset about it
➤ be alone for days accepting whomever comes without making any claims or taking them for granted
➤ lose something you have planned without bitter tears
➤ begin to 'understand' the person who does not understand you
➤ learn the rhythm of an elderly person, even if you are not one yourself
➤ learn to 'listen' with the ears of your soul to the murmurs of someone suffering silently
➤ live the inescapable present moment.

Getting up

I emerge from sleep with one overpowering sensation: pain.

I listen. I listen to my aching body...It is like this every morning. It is the first thing that greets me when my mind has not yet become aware of the rest of the world. I do not feel refreshed...I would love not to do anything, in the vain hope that I will regain my strength and relieve this pain. But I really must get up and take the first dose of medication. My body won't function without it. I cannot lean on my elbow, my back hurts and my joints – almost every one – would like to go on strike...Now is the high point. Transferring on to the wheelchair...I do not think I am going to manage...I grit my teeth...I have managed. I am exhausted but now I can begin the day.

Futility

Is it possible that suffering will not end for me in this world?

…My brain is a total blank. I feel that I have suffered all these years for nothing. It seems absurd to pray. I feel a strange emptiness inside…I am not desperate or distressed. It is just that I am fully aware of the level of destruction in my body and…I do not understand any more…

Why am I still living? Why have other people died without as many years of suffering as I have had? Why do I still have to suffer? Sometimes, I am so tired that I imagine that my death will be truly liberating. You know how much I love life but, it is hard…

Essential thing

I remember something that happened to me during one of my countless hospital admissions. I felt unwell and I rang the bell to call someone. One of my colleagues came and I only managed to say to her, 'I don't feel well, but I don't know how to explain what is wrong. I only feel that I am not well.'

She called the duty doctor who came quickly. He looked the situation over and went off almost without saying a word.

Usually when I do not feel well my natural inclination is to be alone, but that moment I needed him to wait. Just a brief question, 'How are you?' Just a brief touch of my hand, a tap on my shoulder, to make me understand that he was there with me, engaging in my suffering. Just a few words before going away such as, 'I can't stop. I must go away to understand what is happening to you…' That would have been enough.

Instead, as often happens with healthcare workers, they are convinced that they have already done 'enough' so they escape as soon as they have done the necessary. They go off, and you do not give the essential thing. It only takes a brief moment to say to the patient, 'I am here.' In that moment you feel loved and regarded as a person and not like a number or a diagnosis.

Better acquainted

On one side, there is you with your strength and on the other side we with our weakness.

You with your enthusiasm, and we with our seeming resignation.

You with your haste, and we with our enforced patience.

You with your thoughts on life, we with our acceptance of the daily reality we live.

You with your struggle, at times, to find a relationship with the Absolute and we who have the Absolute within us.

You with your fear of suffering and we who are suffering embodied.

You with your 'whys' and we who are an unfathomable response for you.

You who always make plans for the future and we whose future is 'now'.

You who can allow yourself the luxury of not asking while we are forced to do so…

What do you think? Wouldn't it be worthwhile beginning to be better 'acquainted' – from the 'inside'?

Advice to a doctor

From a letter to a doctor friend.

The profession, which you have chosen, is all-consuming…I have no wish to alarm you! It is just that you are already beginning to speak about demotivated trainee doctors and specialists! May I say something?

They tried to get rid of some of my 'sentimental' – according to some of my colleagues – ideas as soon as I had finished nursing school. Apart from one occasion, they were not successful. The patient has always been at the centre for me and comes first. The night shift was especially demanding for me. I would do several rounds because I realised that often the patients do not ring the bell because they are afraid of disturbing you. During the night – and it is very long if you are unwell – there are infinite opportunities to 'listen' and garner 'souls' (you know what I mean, don't you?). It is not always easy. In fact, compared with when I was nursing, today's nurses have ten times more to do. Understaffing, the dreadful shifts and work that often goes unrecognised guarantee that, after a while, people take 'shortcuts' to survive. Where mainly? Relationships inevitably. Everything is so computerised now that I would not be surprised if one day a robot appears before the patient with his case notes to take the medical history. I am exaggerating, but you know what it is like…

Please do not let anyone discourage you! Do not let having a career be the ruin of you. It is right to have one, but not at a patient's expense. Try to keep dreaming, even when you are a knowledgeable, university professor sporting a white beard…

I told you that you ran the risk of burn-out. You can have burn-out in two ways. Either you can let others destroy your inner beauty and find yourself left inside with an empty abyss despite your yacht, two villas etc or you can be consumed by your patients. You have to be giving towards your patients in a healthy, balanced way otherwise, you will get burn-out and will not be able to give anything. Patients will give you other kinds of riches.

Testimony

From a letter of the specialist in charge of Chiara's case at the early stages of her illness.

Your trust in the future – a trust so strong-willed almost to the point of obstinacy – irrespective of the source (faith in a merciful God, your strong character, your upbringing or other) in my humble medical opinion has undoubtedly contributed to improving your prognosis. The immunology expert who first confirmed my clinical suspicions gave you a dismal prognosis…

I do not know if faith and will-power can effectively alter the immune system in the natural history of an illness like xxx to any extent. However, I can nonetheless testify that the way you face your illness greatly influences its natural history.

REFERENCES

1 Chiara M. *Crudele, dolcissimo amore*. Milan: San Paolo Edizioni; 2005.
2 Chiara M. *Oscura, luminosissima notte*. Milan: San Paolo Edizioni; 2008.
3 Foresi P. *Conversazioni di filosofia*. Rome: Città Nuova Editrice; 2001.

Index

T - #0668 - 101024 - C0 - 246/174/10 - PB - 9781846191664 - Gloss Lamination